After the First Full Moon in April

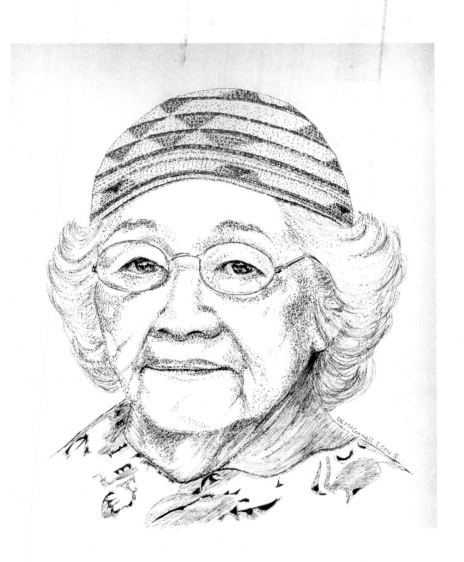

"Josephine Peters in Basketry Cap" by Deborah E. McConnell

After the First Full Moon in April

A Sourcebook of Herbal Medicine from a California Indian Elder

Josephine Grant Peters
and Beverly R. Ortiz

Including contributions from:

Cheryl Beck, Bryan Colegrove, Dwayne Ferris, Patricia Ferris, Zona Ferris,
Wendy Ferris George, LaVerne Glaze, Holly Hensher, Jennifer L. Kalt, Darlene Marshall,
Deborah E. McConnell, Kathleen McCovey, Quetta Peters, Tamara Peters, Ken Wilson

Karuk Plant Names by James A. Ferrara, © Karuk Tribe of California

Left Coast Press Inc.

Walnut Creek, CA

**Left
Coast
Press**
Inc.

Left Coast Press, Inc.
1630 North Main Street, #400
Walnut Creek, California 94596
http://www.lcoastpress.com

Hardback ISBN 978-1-59874-364-7
Paperback ISBN 978-1-61132-791-5
eISBN 978-1-61132-792-2

Library of Congress Cataloging-in-Publication Data

Peters, Josephine Grant.
   After the first full moon in April : a sourcebook of herbal medicine from a California Indian elder / Josephine Grant Peters and Beverly R. Ortiz ; including contributions from Cheryl Beck ... [et al.].
      p. cm.
   Includes bibliographical references.
   ISBN 978-1-59874-364-7 (hardcover : alk. paper)
   ISBN 978-1-61132-791-5 (paperback : alk. paper)
1. Karok Indians--Medicine--California. 2. Herbs--Therapeutic use--California. 3. Karok women--California--Biography. 4. Indian women healers--California--Biography. 5. Karok Indians--California--Social life and customs. I. Ortiz, Bev. II. Beck, Cheryl. III. Title.
   E99.K25P48 2009
   979.4'1004975--dc22

                              2009036627

Printed in the United States of America

The paper used in this publication meets the minimum requirements of American National Standard for Information Sciences—Permanence of Paper for Printed Library Materials, ANSI/NISO Z39.48–1992.

Cover design by Cheryl Carrington
Cover art: "Peppernut Girl," by Lyn Risling

NOTICE: The information in this book is primarily for reference and education. It is not intended to be a substitute for advice of a physician. The authors and editors do not advocate self-diagnosis or self-medication; they urge anyone with continuing symptoms, however minor, to seek medical advice. The reader should be aware that any plant substance, whether used as food or medicine, externally or internally, may cause an allergic reaction in some people.

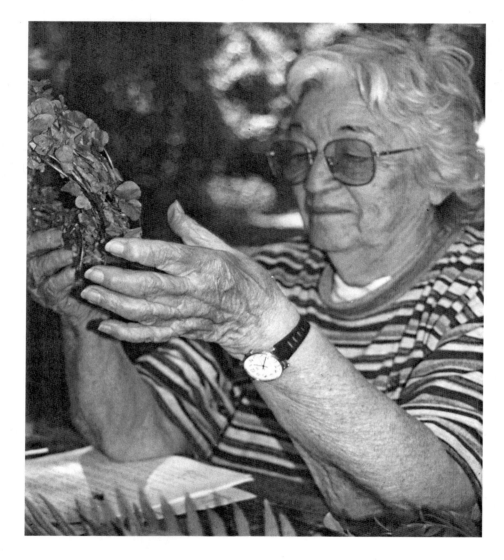

Josephine describes the uses of "tea" (yerba buena), which she had previously bundled into a ring, then dried, for storage. Photo by Beverly Ortiz.

For Bryan Colegrove (Hupa/Yurok/Karuk), Kathy McCovey (Karuk), Bradley Marshall (Karuk/Hupa), and Virgil McLaughlin (Karuk/Hupa, 1955–2009), with thanks for the assistance they provide by taking me out to gather plants, and by gathering plants for me.

JOSEPHINE PETERS

For Josephine, whose knowledge, generosity, and patient, good nature, made it all possible.

BEVERLY R. ORTIZ

CONTENTS

Preface, *Beverly Ortiz* | 9

Acknowledgments, *Beverly Ortiz* | 15

Spirit People, *Darlene Marshall* | 21

The Peppernut, *Josephine Peters* | 23

The Peppernut Story, *Vivien Hailstone, as retold by Darlene Marshall* | 25

1. A Life Well Lived, *Beverly Ortiz* | 27

2. Gathering Ethics, *Jennifer L. Kalt with Bryan Colegrove and Kathleen McCovey* | 67

3. Herbal Medicines and Native Plant Foods | 71

4. The Plants | 99

5. Non-herbal Cures | 197

Endnotes | 199

References | 201

Plant Index | 207

Medical Conditions Index | 213

Subject Index | 217

This book exists because of the strong conviction of herbalist Josephine Grant Peters (Karuk/Shasta/Abenaki) that in order for plants to heal, their medicinal uses must be shared. When Josephine and I first discussed this book, I asked her how much information she wanted to publish about the plants. When I asked that question, I was thinking about the innumerable ethnobotanies that have been published that do not include information about how medicinal plants are gathered and processed, or about the dosages that should be given to treat particular illnesses. When asked about this, Josephine was resolute that preparation details and dosages should indeed be included, with the exception of a handful of plants that she felt were so inherently dangerous to use that the details of their use should only be shared with local tribal people. The focus here is medicinal and food use. The spiritual purposes for which the Karuk use plants will remain with the Karuk community.

Although Josephine's collaboration with me and several other individuals in the creation of this book is certainly an act of tremendous generosity, Josephine herself would not see it in these terms. She wants to preserve plant knowledge for the benefit of future generations, but the level of detail in this book is motivated by something much more profound—Josephine's immutable conviction that unless she shares this information, the ability that she and other people have to heal others with these plants will spiritually die.

In making the decision to share her plant knowledge in a book, Josephine considered the fact that there are many people today who lack the type of restraint that was inherent in the way her people approached the gathering of plants for millennia; today there are people and companies who harvest these plants without any thought of giving back for what they take or of the overall sustainability of the plant populations. Josephine has witnessed the damage that unethical gatherers have done to particular patches of particular plants; but still, the plants will not heal if the knowledge is not shared. So a chapter on gathering ethics has been included in this book to guide people in sustainable plant gathering.

The plant knowledge in this book reflects the whole of Josephine's life. While some readers who seek to find in this book a frozen-in-time explication of ancient Karuk plant uses may be disappointed, the Karuk have never lived a frozen-in-time existence, separated from other people. A considerable portion of the plant uses in this book are based on ancestral practices, as shared with Josephine by members of her extended family and several community elders, but much of it is also based on the type of plant uses that one might come across in any relatively isolated, late 1920s and early 1930s rural community, where doctors trained in modern medicine lived miles away and hospitals were not an option.

When Josephine was young, she heard the dynamite explosions that signaled the conversion of dirt roads suitable for pack trains into paved roads suitable for cars and trucks. Josephine knew a bit of the world that preceded the pack trains, when foot trails linked one distant, small community to another, and river crossings occurred in redwood dugouts, but she never lived in that world.

The larger world began to intrude into Karuk country some seventy years before Josephine was born, in the 1850s during the gold rush, and many of Josephine's plant uses reflect the knowledge and sensibilities about plant use that the newcomers brought with them. They also reflect the knowledge and sensibilities of people Josephine met as she moved throughout California before settling in the Hoopa Valley, and later as she traveled throughout the United States and beyond. For this reason, the plant knowledge shared by Josephine within these pages includes uses of plants she learned from the sons of a Chinese herbalist and American Indian and indigenous doctors she met at conferences and other events throughout the United States and internationally. It also includes Josephine's own sensibilities about how to use particular plants that are based on her own experience trying them herself and later prescribing them to others.

Because this is a very personal ethnobotany, rooted in the knowledge of a particular woman from a particular place with a particular history, the book begins with a detailed summary of Josephine's life, contextualized within the broader framework of Karuk culture and history, the history of Josephine's immediate ancestors, and Josephine's wide-ranging interactions with other tribal people both in the region of her Somes Bar birthplace and further afield. The plant listings that form the core of this book are further contextualized with information about how Josephine learned the uses of particular plants and about the several levels on which she thinks about and uses plants. There is information about the spiritual and practical contexts of that use, as well as information about how the plants were, and continue to be, managed with specialized burning, digging, and pruning techniques that enhance their growth.

From the perspective of outsiders who know nothing about the history of northwest California and nothing about the plants, Josephine Grant Peters will seem like the extraordinary human being that she is. But Josephine sees herself as a very ordinary human being. Josephine would be the first to tell you that what she has accomplished in her life is no more extraordinary than what innumerable individuals of her generation and life experience have accomplished, so she would not wish to be singled for out what she has done. To ensure that people understand this, the life history chapter of this book includes the cultural involvements of Josephine's peers and the mutual support and inspiration they have provided to each other. Family, community, and place have always been important in Josephine's world, and they remain as fundamental today as they were thousands of years ago.

Josephine's own words have been incorporated into the text in italic typeface. Her voice is intended to remind you that this is a very personal ethnobotany, one which represents a lifetime of learning and thinking about plants and of taking and

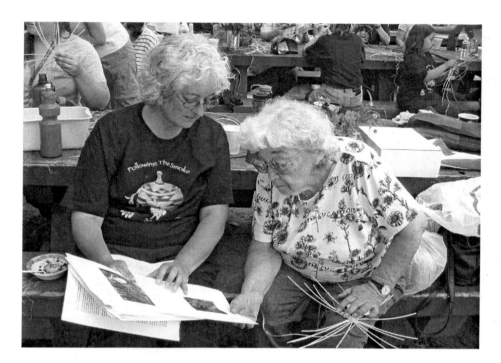

Beverly Ortiz and Josephine Peters at Following the Smoke, Camp Creek, west of Orleans, California, discussing a draft of this book, and reviewing photographs for inclusion. Photo by Nancy Cussary, July 14, 2005.

prescribing plant remedies by a particular woman with a particular history. Hopefully, Josephine's words will help you access the utter joy I have had in traveling with her through the landscape she knows so intimately, learning about the plants firsthand. I hope that a small measure of Josephine's inestimable good humor, practicality, forthrightness, and generosity will also shine through.

My role in this book has been to document and write down Josephine's life history and plant knowledge. Josephine shared this knowledge with me in much the same way that she learned—through experience, conversation, stories, and the serendipity of the moment. While I conducted several formal, audio-taped interviews with Josephine about the plants, much of what I learned was revealed as we sat around the kitchen table and chatted, visited at cultural events, and traveled together to find particular plants, or simply traveled to the market or a wedding. We did not discuss a given plant and all its uses in a fill-in-the-blank chronology. Instead, uses, preparation details, and dosages unfolded across several years in the ebb and flow of conversation, and in an ebb and flow of questions that I asked to clarify and amplify the details. The list of plants that Josephine uses grew in the manner of those plants, gradually and steadily, nurtured by previous generations, and supported by the present one. Like the plants, the entire project was nurtured and supported throughout by numerous people who helped with research and plant identifications, took photographs, and otherwise assisted with the myriad tasks necessary to grow a book. The story of how the book came into being, and the many people who helped with it, is told in the remaining pages of this forward and in the acknowledgments that follow.

I first met Josephine Peters in 1998, when she spoke about medicinal uses of plants at "Following the Smoke," a collaborative volunteer project sponsored by Karuk Indigenous Basketweavers, Six Rivers National Forest, the Bureau of Land

Management, The Karuk Tribe of California, and CalTrans. My presence that day resulted from an invitation from *News from Native California* to cover the first-ever Following the Smoke in 1997. Ken Wilson, Following the Smoke project coordinator and Six Rivers National Forest Heritage Resources program manager, extended the invitation. At the time, I was skills and technology columnist for *News*, and the editor, Jeannine Gendar, asked me if I would like to go and write about the project. I looked forward to the opportunity to learn more about the use of plants by Native peoples in California, an area of particular interest for me since the summer of 1976, when I worked as an oral historian in the Plumas National Forest. Most especially, I anticipated the pleasant camaraderie of time spent talking with weavers and gathering basketry materials.

Following the Smoke was named after a strategy once used by weavers in the Klamath-Trinity River area to track the Forest Service's autumn slash burning program in the hope of finding suitably burned basketry materials (Heffner 1984). In the old days, Native peoples managed the landscape by setting fires in seasonal rounds. These fires kept woodlands and forests open and filled with mature trees; ensured that seed harvests would be plentiful; killed disease organisms that thrive in the duff and decaying debris that accumulate in unburned areas; and readily returned nutrients to the soil. Where fires burned, new sprouts proliferated, which in turn provided food for elk, antelope, and deer. Fire also served as an important tool for basketmakers. In northern California, for instance, fires ensured the growth of straight, supple hazel shoots and robust, pliable beargrass blades.

In short, the fires set by Native peoples helped renew the land, ensuring the health and productivity of the plants and wildlife upon which the people depended for sustenance. After non-Indians outlawed these aeons-old prescribed burning practices, basketmakers had to hope that slash burns had inadvertently done the job or make do with inferior materials.

Today basketmakers in the Klamath-Trinity forests no longer need to rely on the chance of slash burning. Instead, they've worked long and hard to successfully advocate for the prescribed burning of basketry plants on Forest Service lands. Due to staff turnover, however, they must continually educate the general public, land management agency personnel, and in particular, policy makers in those agencies, about these and other issues of concern, such as herbicide spraying of basketry plants, medicines, and food.

The Karuk Indigenous Basketweavers, a group of basketweavers of Karuk heritage, hosted Following the Smoke as part of these wide-ranging educational efforts. This award-winning project, which occurred from 1997–2007, was part of Passport in Time (PIT), a nationwide USDA Forest Service program intended to involve individuals and families in archaeological and historic preservation projects in national forests. Following the Smoke, one of more than a hundred PIT projects offered annually throughout the United States, was the first PIT project to include cultural exchange and policy change as its goal. In addition to learning about local plant use and weaving techniques, volunteers helped gather basketry materials for distribution to elder weavers. They also prepared sites with beargrass and/or hazel for controlled burning in collaboration with the Forest Service and a private landholder, clearing and stacking brush and creating a fire line.[*]

---

[*]For more about Following the Smoke see Ortiz (1998:21-29 and 1999:13-16).

At the 1998 PIT, Josephine expanded participants' awareness of Karuk plant use beyond the realm of baskets by explaining the medicinal properties of innumerable plants growing near the camp. Her repertoire ranged from plant-based cures for burns, sores, blisters, rashes, indigestion, and coughs, to those for kidney stones, stroke, and cancer. She described wormwood's use as a tick repellent when rubbed on one's arms and legs; a decoction of yerba buena for fevers; how trillium (mother-wort) bulbs ease labor pains; and the manner in which Oregon grape root steeped in hot water becomes a blood purifier. Throughout, she interlaced cautionary stories about the destruction of herbal gathering locales through logging activities, herbicide spraying along roadsides, and thoughtless greed:

> When I go out, I just gather what I think I need.... We don't have any ginseng in the area any more.... We used to go up the creek where I live, but they've gathered it all out. They don't leave anything for seed.

If the plants are properly cared for, Josephine emphasized, *There's enough herbs on the earth to cure everything.*

Following the Smoke has been a dynamic, poignant, and joy-filled experience; the weavers' generosity and warmth a great gift. I was blessed to return every year of the project's eleven years, to renew the friendships made, continue documenting the contemporary cultural involvements and policy needs of its indigenous participants, and assist with activities.

In 2001 Ken Wilson phoned me at the request of Wendy Ferris George, Vice Chair of the California Indian Basketweavers Association, to ask if I would take a lead role in an effort to preserve Josephine's cultural knowledge, especially that pertaining to medicinal plant uses. The need to preserve Josephine's knowledge had been on many people's minds, including my own, and Ken successfully applied to the USDA-Forest Service, Pacific Southwest Region, for a grant to do just that. The grant resulted in a Challenge Cost-Share Agreement between the Six Rivers National Forest and the California Indian Basketweavers Association Northwestern Field Office. The Cost-Share Agreement provided an invaluable opportunity to produce an overview of Josephine's life history, identify the plants she uses for medicinal purposes, and describe the illnesses she treats with them.

The current book greatly expands on the information generated by the Challenge Cost-Share Agreement, providing additional information about Josephine's life, as well as detailed instructions about how she processes herbs for medicinal and edible purposes.

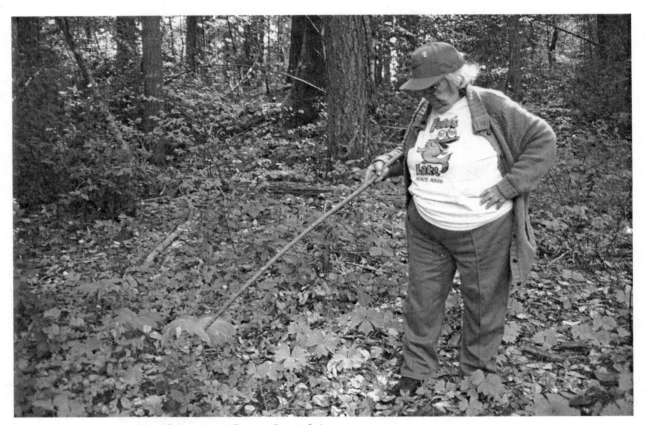

Josephine explains the uses of false Solomon's seal. Photo by Beverly Ortiz.

Our forest is like a drugstore.

JOSEPHINE PETERS
March 10, 2004

That this book could be written at all is due to Josephine's abiding commitment to share her knowledge with a wide audience. Her inestimable generosity, good humor, forthrightness, and practicality have graced the entire undertaking. Her warm hospitality and indefatigable patience carried it forward to completion. Her extensive archive of documents pertaining to local and family history gave a context to the work.

Josephine's daughters were extremely helpful. Cheryl Beck reviewed drafts of the manuscript and provided important guidance. She sent me a copy of a *Siskiyou Pioneer* article written by Frank A. Grant III about the family's history, and a copy of C. Hart Merriam's field notes, edited by Robert Heizer and based on Merriam's interviews with Cheryl's great-grandmother, Ellen Brazille Grant. She also sent me photographs of her great-grandparents, a lovely photograph of her grandparents' ranch, where Josephine was raised, and arranged for her granddaughter Samantha McDonald to write a tribute to Josephine, which Cheryl edited.

Tamara Peters provided much appreciated encouragement and loaned me several family photographs. The stories and reminiscences she shared helped provide a context for and humanity to her mother's life history.

Quetta Peters (Cree) and Jene McCovey (Yurok) provided support and warmhearted hospitality during my many trips to Hoopa. Some years prior to the project's beginning, Quetta compiled a list of plants used by her mom, and what they were used for. This list, along with one made by students at The University of California at Riverside, provided the base upon which the project's plant use information was compiled.

Many thanks, as well, to Josephine's niece Cindy Sylvia (Hoopa/Yurok/Karuk) for her hospitality, good cheer and encouragement.

Darlene Marshall's stunning poetry and prose provides an important context for understanding the spiritual significance of the plants. Darlene (Hupa/Yurok/Karuk) graciously hosted me at her Hoopa Valley home on several occasions, where she regaled me with many compelling stories about the cultural contributions of Josephine, her aunt Vivien Hailstone, and other community elders. These stories provided invaluable perspective for the life history chapter of this work, about which Darlene provided vital feedback. Darlene introduced me to her sister Andrea Kelsey, who also provided important insights about community history and cultural involvements. Darlene's cousin Lyn Risling (Karuk, Yurok, and Member of the Hoopa Tribe) created the beautiful painting, *The Peppernut Story*, which graces the cover of the book, and helps bring that sacred narrative to life.

Quetta Peters, Josephine Peters and Jene McCovey outside their Hoopa Valley home. Photo by Beverly Ortiz, 2001.

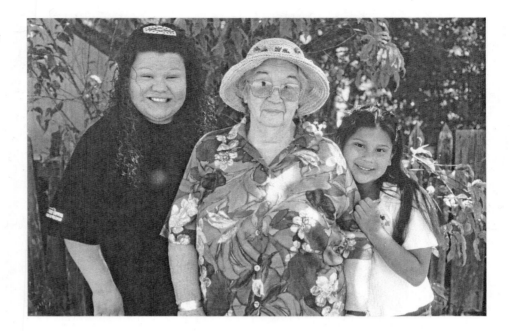

The work was guided throughout by Bryan Colegrove (Hupa/Yurok/Karuk), Dwayne Ferris (Karuk), Patricia Ferris (Hupa/Yurok/Chimariko), Zona Ferris (Karuk), Wendy Ferris George (Hupa/Yurok/Karuk/Chimariko), LaVerne Glaze (Karuk/Yurok), Holly Hensher (Karuk), Jennifer L. Kalt, Deborah E. McConnell (Hupa/Yurok), Kathleen Mc-Covey (Karuk), and Ken Wilson. In addition to the input they provided at several meetings held with Josephine, they helped implement the research and nurtured the project throughout. Their generous efforts have greatly enriched the results.

Bryan Colegrove and Kathy McCovey took Josephine to gather plants, interviewed her about their use, and took notes. When Josephine's health would not permit her to join them, they gathered plants under her direction. In addition, Kathy suggested the title *After the First Full Moon in April* during a brainstorming session with Jo, myself, and several of the other people involved. Kathy gave me a draft of a report she wrote about the history and culture of the Karuk. This formed the basis of the introduction to Karuk history and culture provided in the life history section of this work. Kathy also collaborated with Erin Rentz (Karuk), Frank K. Lake (Karuk), and Luna Latimer Lake on the identification of plants. Frank and Luna took photographs of some plants, as did botanist Sydney Carothers. Stephen W. Edwards, director of the East Bay Regional Park District Botanic Garden at Tilden Regional Park, and Susan Agnew, located several plant photographs in the garden archives. I would also like to thank Steve Edwards and Bert Johnson for reviewing and providing Latin binominals for pressed samples of some of Josephine's herbs.

Patricia and Dwayne Ferris interviewed Josephine about plant uses, especially those with spiritual significance, and also took photographs of plants.

Holly Hensher conducted a cassette-taped interview with Josephine about plant uses, and videotaped her in the field.

Jennifer Kalt, the California Indian Basketweavers Association's (CIBA) resource protection associate in the Northwestern Field Office and a botanist, confirmed the Latin binomials, which follow *The Jepson Manual.* She created a herbarium from

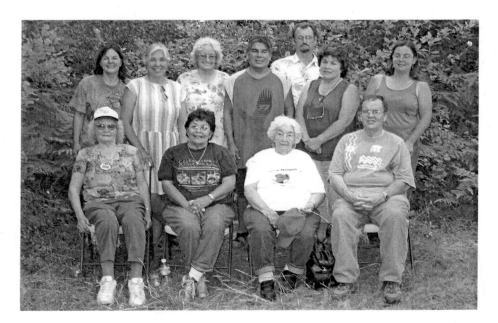

Front row, left to right: Zona Ferris, LaVerne Glaze, Josephine Peters, and Ken Wilson. *Back row, left to right:* Kathy McCovey, Deborah McConnell, Beverly Ortiz, Bryan Colegrove, Dwayne Ferris, Pat Ferris, and Jennifer Kalt. Taken at Camp Creek, near Panámnik (Orleans), California during Following the Smoke. Photo by Sally Jones, July 13, 2005.

plant specimens gathered by herself, Bryan Colegrove, Kathy McCovey, and myself. Jennifer took notes about plant uses and created a computerized, comparative database of Quetta's plant list and that of Riverside. This database revealed a number of plants for which use information had not yet been obtained or confirmed, and inconsistencies in scientific names identified by the Riverside students. It was also used as the basis for a flow chart listing those plants for which photographs and/or specimens had been obtained.

Jennifer wrote Chapter 2, Gathering Ethics, with guidance from Bryan Colegrove and Kathy McCovey. She photographed plants growing in the field, and accompanied Jo, myself, and an interested college student on an excursion from Hoopa, nearly to Redding, to document some of the plants. Jennifer later made her laptop available to me for compiling additional information during another visit with Jo. Jennifer made that same laptop available in 2005, when we made editorial changes to the manuscript at the 2005 Following the Smoke, first by daylight, then by candlelight and Coleman Lantern light while seated at a picnic table. Additionally, Jennifer scanned the project's slide collection and videotaped Bryan Colegrove talking about Josephine's importance in his life. Deborah McConnell, Director of CIBA's Northwestern Field Office, administered the Cost-Share Agreement between CIBA and Six Rivers National Forest that funded initial research about Josephine's use of plants growing within the forest area. She interviewed Josephine about plant uses and took meticulous notes and photographs of Josephine and certain plants. She also drew the elegant illustration of Josephine in her basket cap.

The following people participated in and documented Josephine's salve making process at Deborah's Hoopa Valley home on March 10, 2004: Bryan Colegrove, Kathy McCovey, and Virgil McLauglin gathered the herbs; Zona Ferris and Jennifer Kalt made written notes; Jennifer Kalt and Bryan Colegrove made videotapes; and LaVerne Glaze and Deborah McConnell took still photographs. Pat Ferris, Holly Hensher, and Quetta Peters joined them in learning about salve making.

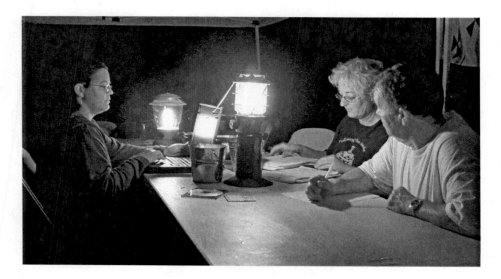

Beverly Ortiz, Ken Wilson, and Jennifer Kalt working on the book by lantern light at Following the Smoke, Camp Creek, California, July 13, 2005. Photo courtesy unknown Following the Smoke participant.

Language specialist James A. Ferrara compiled and edited the Karuk names listed in the text in consultation with Karuk elder Violet Super and linguist William Bright. He also consulted the writings of linguist J. P. Harrington. Those found here are excerpted from draft four of a manuscript in Jim's possession, "Scientific (Latin) Designations for Plants, with Corresponding Karuk Names," completed March 8, 2004, and a second manuscript, "Plant and Animal Names Composite List with English Glosses of Karuk Terms." The Karuk Tribe of California holds the copyright to this material.

In addition to Cheryl Beck and Tamara Peters, Holly Hensher, Jennifer Kalt, Deborah McConnell, Kathy McCovey, and Ken Wilson reviewed and commented on drafts of the manuscript.

Jeannine Gendar, Heyday Books editorial director, provided valuable advice about scanning images for publication. Many thanks to Annamarie Guerrero and Jennifer Kalt for their assistance with scanning numerous prints and slides, respectively; as well as to Cecilia Perez, who helped select images from Josephine's photo albums.

Most of the projects' archives will be deposited with Humboldt State University's Indian Natural Resources Science and Engineering Program. The plant specimens will be deposited in HSU's Herbarium.

It has been my honor and utter joy to work with Josephine and everyone else involved in bringing the project to completion. I had the great fortune to share oral history techniques with project members, compile the data contributed by them, and conduct extensive cassette-taped and written interviews with Jo about her life and plant use. Along the way, I took still photographs of Jo with her children, giving presentations and gathering plants, of the plants themselves, the processing of the herbs, historic family photographs, and baskets and other objects made by Jo. We traveled to look at plants and document their uses on several occasions. Once, we spent the day traveling with Jene McCovey to look at, photograph, and discuss places along the Trinity and Klamath Rivers that were important to Jo in her childhood and later life.

I used Quetta's list and that of Riverside as the basis for asking Jo detailed questions about every plant, including preparation and dosage information. As the list of plants steadily expanded beyond these initial, vital compilations, the awe I felt when I first heard Jo discuss plant uses in 1998 continued to increase. That sense of awe grew as I reviewed notes, transcribed tapes and compiled the plant information,

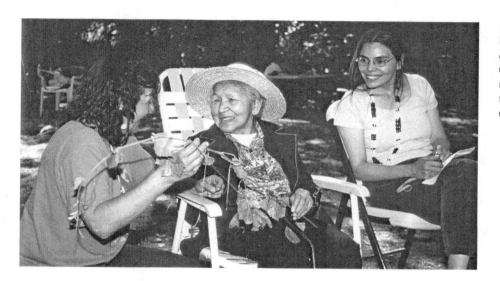

Left to right: Kathy McCovey, Violet Super and Susan Gehr, language director, Karuk Tribe of California, discussing the Karuk name for wild grape at Following the Smoke. Photograph by Beverly Ortiz, ca. July 2006.

leading me to ask additional questions to fill in the details. It occurred anew as I reviewed and copied documents in Josephine's extensive archives. The process of writing it all down renewed my awe, and my gratitude, again and again.

During numerous visits and telephone calls to refine and expand upon the information shared within the growing compendium, the clarity and consistency with which Josephine recalled the details was both gratifying and astonishing. Although in the final years of the project Josephine's health precluded her from traveling into the field to view the plants, she was able to review color photographs downloaded by me from CalPhotos to ensure the accuracy of the plant identifications, as well as review plant specimens brought to her by Kathy McCovey and Bryan Colegrove.

During the course of this project, Zona Ferris and LaVerne Glaze shared their own knowledge of plant use with me. This very important information, along with that shared by Frank Scott, will be published at a later date in another venue.

Much appreciation goes to Joe and Carol J. Ellick, whom I met at the 2007 Following the Smoke, where a draft of the manuscript was shared with participants. Joe and Carol introduced me to Mitch Allen, publisher of Left Coast Press, who immediately recognized the value of the information contained within this book, and agreed to publish it. Since then, Jennifer Collier, Senior Editor of Left Coast Press, has ably overseen the myriad tasks necessary to bring this work into publication. I very much appreciate Jennifer's keen eye for detail, nuance and context. Her editorial suggestions have greatly enriched the results, as has the skillful copy editing of Nathalie Arnold, whose sensitivity to the material, and expertise in the finer details of grammar, phrasing, and format, brought consistency to the content, while maintaining its overall tone. I would like to extend many thanks to proofreader Sally Gregg, whose passion for the English language, and sensitivity to the written word, resulted in a superbly-polished book. Finally, I would like to recognize the talented work of Lisa Devenish of Devenish Design. Lisa brought immense heart and beauty to the overall appearance of the book, reflecting in her design the heart and beauty of Josephine herself.

On behalf of myself, Josephine, and the project contributors, I would like to thank Mitch, Jennifer, and the entire Left Coast Press team for helping Josephine fulfill her dream of sharing the healing qualities of plants with the broader world.

Beverly Ortiz

Spirit People

Darlene Marshall (Hupa/Yurok/Karuk), 2004

In the beginning, before there was anything, there was God.
Later, there were the Spirit People, and animals could talk.

One day, God said, "It is time for people. We must make the world
ready for them. First they will need things to eat so that they can live.
The animals will be food and we will fill the water with fish.
Plants, trees, and almost everything made can be used by the people.

We will not make it easy. To some animals we will give the gift of speed,
some will have great strength, and some keen eyesight. We will be a part
of every living thing and each will have the gift of survival."

So it was done. The Spirit People became part of every living thing. Some
spirits became birds, some lived in rocks to keep the memory of everything that
happens, and some lived in the plants. There was much discussion about which
spirit would become which plant. Some spirit people knew that useful objects
such as baskets would also be very beautiful. Others wanted to be acorn
trees because people would depend on them. The greatest care was given
in choosing who would have the honor of being medicinal plants. "This was
important," God said, "because when the people get sick they will need this,
our greatest gift. But all plants are important and must be shown respect."

The people came and learned the importance of all God's gifts. They learned
that all living things are to be respected. Some learned to use plants to make life
easier and some were gifted with the knowledge of plant use for healing. When
the people were sick, they thanked Creator God for this, the greatest gift.

We burn root and pray.

We think good thoughts and weave.

We grind our acorns to feed our family.

We sing as we rock the baby in the basket.

It is good that we live here in this place

that the Creator made for us.

Thank you, Spirit People.

Thank you Creator God.

The Peppernut

Josephine Peters, 2001

A long time ago, when they had the brush dances . . . they'd say the little peppernut used to go out and roll around in front of the crowd to try to let people know she had medicine. Now we use the peppernut. We crack them, and we use the little nut inside for a lot of things. We can use it for healing diabetic sores, bedsores, any kind of ulcerated sore, impetigo, boils. It'll draw blood poisoning. . . . It's an old Indian tale, and it told that the peppernut was good for a lot of things . . . Vivien [Hailstone] used to tell it.

The Peppernut Story

Vivien Hailstone (Yurok/Karuk/Member of the Hoopa Tribe),
as retold by Darlene Marshall, 2004

Not everyone could be a medicine woman. One had to train for many years and come before the most knowledgeable one for the test. In our story, there is a mouse, a frog, and a peppernut in training.

The mouse came before The-One-Who-Was-There and said, "I have been working very hard to meet the test."

"Indeed you have," The-One-Who-Was-There replied. "There is something about you that I have noticed also. You have a very long nose. It starts high in your forehead and ends out over your chin. That is very well, however, for this is the way that you are."

Next came the frog. "You have seen the training that I have been going through," she said.

"Yes," said The-One-Who-Was-There. "You have been studying the ways with great care. There is something I have noticed about you however. You are covered with bumps. They cover much of your body. That is very well, however, for that is the way that you are."

Now it was time for the little peppernut to come before The-One-Who-Was-There. Others who had failed to pass the test said to her, "You will never become a medicine woman. You don't have legs."

"Oh," cried the little peppernut, as tears came to her eyes.

They said, "You don't have any arms either." Feeling so bad, the peppernut began to dance, and she cried. She rolled back and forth before The-One-Who-Was-There, rolling this way and that, crying and singing her little song.

When the choice was made, it was the peppernut maiden who passed the test and became the medicine woman. The peppernut leaves are still used in religious ceremonies today.

CHAPTER ONE

A Life Well Lived[1]

AT HOME

A white picket fence protects the herbs, flowers, and fruit trees that Josephine Peters has planted in her Hoopa Valley yard. Inside the gate, the dog and cats offer an expectant greeting. Behind the house, an eclectic variety of chickens provide fresh eggs. Herbs hang upside down, drying, inside the enclosed porch.

Immediately inside the door of Josephine's home, a display case filled with basketry medallions, beadwork, pottery, and other local creations beckons, while the woodstove opposite warms the living room and much of the rest of the house in cold weather. In the kitchen, beading supplies and basketry materials are stored at the ready. Letters, invitations, and basketry and beadwork projects commonly adorn the kitchen table, as do boxes packed with Josephine's latest creations, ready for mailing to park and museum gift shops throughout the state and beyond. Additional sales items, meant for drop-in buyers or sales at events, are boxed nearby.

Josephine's day starts early and ends late. In the morning, she gardens and tends to the chickens, takes care of household chores, sees her youngest, Jene McCovey (Yurok), off to school, and reads the paper. She works on the daily crossword puzzle, often filling it in entirely, other times, missing only a few words. Visitors come and go throughout the day and into the evening—family members and friends to say hello, visit, and assist in the yard; friends and relatives bringing gifts of local fruit, vegetables, fish, venison, basketry materials, and herbs; nieces and nephews helping to prepare the fruit and vegetables for canning; locals and others from greater distances seeking medical advice; and tribal artisans with newly created jewelry for sale.

Day and night, Josephine tends to myriad phone calls and monitors local news on a police scanner. When she can't attend in person, she listens with rapt attention to the tribal radio station's broadcast of the home team basketball game.

Often, Josephine can be found at points near and distant sharing her herbal and other cultural knowledge at diverse public events and at schools with students of all ages; enjoying family and friends at reunions, birthday parties, and other special occasions; participating in community events and activities; attending ceremonies; or demonstrating basketry and selling culturally inspired jewelry at a variety of shows and gatherings.

In addition to the daily ebb and flow of Josephine's activities, there is a seasonal ebb and flow. After winter's high river waters, and before the onset of spring, it's time to gather river roots for basketry. Early spring is the optimal time to gather gray willow and hazel "sticks" for basketry, just as the leaves begin to form.

The gathering of most medicinal herbs takes place after the first full moon in April, when their "strength" is greatest. Other herbs, like yarrow, ceanothus, St. John's wort, and redwood sorrel, are gathered after they bloom.

April is the best time to gather alder bark, ceanothus (soapbrush), and Douglas fir for basketry. May through June is the time to gather "black fern," " (aka five-finger fern) another basketry material, and May the optimal time for angelica. Durango root achieves a "good color" for basketry dye in spring, which is also the time to make medicinal salves, when the herbs are "fresh."

In early June, canning commences with the ripening of the cherry crop. It continues through July and August to include a variety of fruits, garden vegetables, fish, and elk and deer meat. October is huckleberry gathering season, while October and November are the months to gather woodwardia for basketry, and acorns and peppernuts for food and medicine. Following the rains, mushroom harvesting commences, as does the digging of pine and spruce roots for basketry.

In 2004, Bryan Colegrove (Hupa/Yurok), reflecting on his many visits with Josephine, described the values she exemplifies and the importance of elders, family, and community in the day-to-day lives of the Karuk, Yurok, and Hupa peoples.

I'm the oldest of nine kids. My dad was a hunter and fisherman and provided for the elders. We'd go around and give deer meat and salmon to those who couldn't get it. Josephine was married to one of my uncles, and we came over and visited. She's always been special. We brought fish and deer meat. If someone was sick, we'd ask for medicines and get something from her.

I left the area to work in Colorado, Texas, and Oregon. After I moved back in the 1980s, I started going around doing what my dad and grandfather did. I started visiting more with Auntie Jo. She was having a hard time getting around, so I'd take her some of the plants. I'd get deer meat, smoked, fresh, and canned salmon, eels, acorns, seaweed, surf fish, mussels, shells, spruce root, everything we utilize. I'd go down and gather in Mendocino, Humboldt and Del Norte Counties. If anybody needs anything, we're always sharing. If somebody needs help, you can't say no. You've got to be respectful. Respect the land and plants. (Personal communication with Jennifer Kalt, 2004)

KARUK CULTURE AND HISTORY

Josephine Peters is Karuk by birth and upbringing, although her heritage is also Konimuhu (Shasta), a neighboring group, and Rouge River, Abenaki, from the northeastern United States. Josephine has deep bonds—socially, communally, and by marriage—to the Yurok and Hupa. She has lived most of her life within the homeland of the Hupa, along the upper Trinity River, in the verdant and expansive, five-mile-long Hoopa Valley. The cultures of the Karuk, Yurok, and Hupa are nearly the same, although all three peoples spoke, as some continue to speak, entirely distinct languages—part of the Hokan, Algonkian, and Athapascan language families (see Figure 1.1) (Bright 1978: 180; Pilling 1978: 137; Wallace 1978: 164).

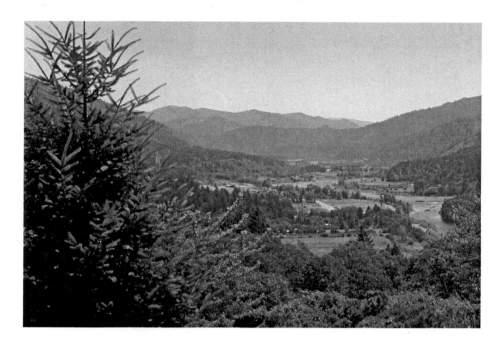

Figure 1.1.
View of the Hoopa Valley. Photo
by Beverly Ortiz.

The homeland of the Karuk is part of the ruggedly stunning, glacier- and river-carved places now known as the Siskiyou Mountains, Marble Mountains, and Salmon-Trinity Alps (Bell 1991: 20–26; Bright 1978: 180). The Karuk lived, and continue to live, in a world animated by spirits. As explained by Karuk author Julian Lang (1994: 22–24):

> Ikxaréeyav means God in the People's language, and refers both to our many spirit-deities, and nowadays, to the monotheistic God of modern religions. We have deified everything in the natural world. We consider all of nature to be alive, possessing both feelings and a consciousness. Hence the natural world is capable of seeing and hearing us, "blessing" us, and taking pity on us. The Earth is a physical manifestation of God's creative spirit, and we, Human Beings, are recognized by the earth as a part of the natural world. ... Our sense is that all of nature grows from the Earth as strands of long hair connecting the present with the beginning of time and original knowledge.
>
> ... The Ikxaréeyavs were hyper-alive, meaning their lives were purely creative. Each moment of their existence resulted in some kind of creation: the realization of a natural law, a powerful song, or a healing herb and medicine formula to cure the gravest ill. The Earth itself was new when they were alive. And, like a new love, every moment, every movement, every idea and feeling was without precedent.[2]

As further explained by Kathy McCovey, also Karuk:

> When the Karuk people came into the land, the spirit people taught the Karuk how to live, where to live, what to do and how to do it. When the spirit people knew that the Karuk knew how to live upon the land, the spirit people left the land to the Karuk. When the spirit people left, some of them went up into the sky; some went down into the earth; and some went into the rocks, the trees, the water, and the animals. When the Karuk people go out into the forest, they

are never alone. They are surrounded by the spirit people who taught them how to live upon the land. (Personal communication with Beverly Ortiz, July 27, 2009)

The Karuk social world centered on extended family; their political life on the village where they lived, each one located on dozens of flats extending along some eighty-two miles of the Klamath River, and some two miles of the Salmon River, including Three Dollar Bar, where Josephine Peters grew up. The Karuk homeland extended well beyond these village locations, into the mountains, and several miles up the Salmon River. Villages had some five to thirty semi-subterranean plank houses, one per family, and several sweathouses. Houses were the province of women, visited by men during the two daily meals at dawn and dusk; sweathouses were the province of men, a place where they reached decisions about legal matters, made "hunting medicine," and slept. "Together these two houses," explains Julian Lang, "were at the center of our culture and identity" (1994: 22).

Objects of daily use included elegantly woven baskets, carefully chipped obsidian knives and arrow points, elaborately carved cooking paddles and wooden spoons, meticulously fashioned, bowltube iris-fiber nets, and buoyant redwood dugouts purchased from the Yurok. Abalone pendants, engraved dentalia shells,[3] iridescent pileated woodpecker and mallard featherwork, beargrass braids, and gray pine nut beads adorned ceremonial regalia (Bright 1978: 183–184; Kelly 1930; Lang 1994: 15–22).

The Karuk procured some of their most important foods from the river, upslope fir forests, and oak groves: salmon, deer, and tanoak acorns. They smoked, dried, roasted, or otherwise processed eels, elk, bear, small mammals, and birds and variously pounded, stone boiled, parched, and roasted bulbs, seeds, greens, and nuts.

The modern concept of an uncultivated wild, or wilderness, negates the very different, thousands-of-years-old human relationship between the Karuk, plants, other animal species, and place. It was through this relationship that they managed and reshaped their homeland with such horticultural techniques as burning that enhanced some species, while suppressing others. Although today it is nearly impossible to know exactly what that managed landscape looked like in 1850, when non-Indians intruded, we can get a strong sense of its appearance through the reminiscences of tribal elders, early photographs, and local fire records. In 1997, Ramona Starritt (Karuk), then age 92, described one such managed landscape in the mountainous regions of the Klamath River near Orleans and Happy Camp, before the fire suppression policies of the U.S. Forest Service were implemented:

The Indians burned all over. ... The earlier years it would just burn, burn, burn, until the sun looked like a big orange. It just burned itself out. That was that. They did it for the purpose of their basket weaving, and for the animals. The deer had to eat. They ate the young sprouts. And you could see for miles. You weren't hemmed in with brush. ...

The trees were not hurt in any way. No burns, or anything, because the vegetation was not so high as it is now. ... You go to where the Indians lived and burned, you'll see really tall fir trees. And pine trees and madrone trees were large. ... The change came when the highways came in. ... That was in the late twenties. ...

[E]very fall they burned. You didn't have any brush. ... A lot of times it didn't burn too long, because it was clean [of organic debris]. Nothing to burn.

And it didn't hurt the trees. You go to any old Indian ranch, you'll see the trees tall and healthy looking. [….] When I was young, you could see clear across the gorge. … See a bear climbing up the mountain, or a deer, or anything. (Personal communication with Beverly Ortiz, August 28, 1997)

Burning had several purposes (Lake 2007). As described by Hotelling (1978: 15–16):

The immediate objective was a productive forest assuring an ample supply of food and materials. The fire, controlled as it was, burned off the debris which no longer served a purpose, making it easy to gather the acorns and, interestingly enough, the food so gathered was shared with the wildlife. … Likewise in gathering the huckleberry, both for current and winter use, the bushes here again became large and mature and were burned which gave them young growth and a better quality berry and here again the food was shared with the animals of the forest, particularly the bear.

In addition to burning techniques, the Karuk used, and continue to use, the same horticultural methods that gardeners use in their yards: judicious harvesting, cultivation (digging), pruning, weeding, and debris clearing. Today, Karuk weavers sometimes use coppicing, the cutting back of plants during dormancy to within inches of the ground surface, as a second-best alternative to burning.

Judicious harvesting centers on prohibitions against taking more than can be processed and used. As Virginia Larson (Karuk) has expressed it:

You never ever take more than what you use. If you take something, you use it, and prepare it. … You may have to go out days later and get it again, but don't take a bunch and then not use it. I don't know if it's true, but it was always told to us, "If you do that then bad luck comes." (Personal communication with Beverly Ortiz, August 29, 1997)

Cultivation (digging), weeding, and debris clearing occurred simultaneously whenever the Karuk harvested bulbs, corms, or other underground plant structures. By cultivating the same plants on an annual cycle in the same locales, the Karuk loosened and aerated the soil, improved wintertime soil drainage, increased moisture absorption, and created the conditions that allowed plant tracts to expand.

Pruning increases the vigor and productivity of the plants while stimulating the growth of long, straight, unbranched, flexible, healthy, newborn shoots. It controls insect larvae infestations in particular plants.

Burning results in the growth of pliable, straight, long new shoots of shrubs and other plants, harvested for basketry materials or other purposes. It returns nutrients to the soil, eliminates unhealthy plants, reduces pests, and keeps understory vegetation sufficiently spaced, ensuring that each plant will get the optimum light, water, and nutrients. According to Elsie Griffin, (Yurok) "[Burning] wasn't just done for the gatherers. It was done for the good of the forest" (personal communication with Beverly Ortiz, June 30, 1991).

Beargrass (*Xerophyllum tenax*) provides an apt example of the effects of burning. In northwest California, beargrass, a type of native lily with grasslike blades, provides a yellowish-white overlay in baskets. In the absence of burning, the blades of this plant grow sharp-edged, thick, and brittle. Even when soaked, such blades lack pliability, and the resultant baskets have an uneven, "lumpy" appearance.

Burning converts the previous year's dry blades into nutrient-rich ash and stimulates the growth of supple new blades. The most pliable, longest blades grow in the partial shade of trees, where burning prevents fuel buildup. After curing (drying) and trimming (sizing), such blades lay flatter on the basket's surface than those growing in full sun.

In the old days, the Karuk and Yurok set fires as they moved from the high country, where summer storms occurred, to lower elevations. Such fires, set on a regular basis, kept dry, flammable duff, brush, and other debris from accumulating. Now, because of decades of fire suppression, before a fire can be set, the site must be prepared by clearing brush and logs, creating fire breaks, and measuring for optimum humidity, wind, and air temperature.

Not only do the Karuk manage basketry and other plants at particular times of the year, they harvested them at particular times of the year, which varied with elevation and fluctuations in climate. Karuk, Yurok, and Hoopa weavers, for instance, gather black (aka five-finger) fern (Adiantum aleuticum) stems, used for a black overlay, in late May through the first part of August, depending on the elevation. If gathered too early, the stems will break from lack of firmness; if gathered too late, they will break from brittleness. Spruce (*Picea sitchensis)* root harvesting generally takes place in November, when the roots attain their greatest strength and pliability (Ortiz 1998, 1999).

The objects the Karuk used, and continue to use, while both alluring and useful, contain a deeper meaning when considered within the whole of their cultural context. Beyond the tangible acts of hunting and fishing, or gathering or processing of plant materials, each object resulted from a thousands-of-years-old relationship among people, creation, place, plants, and animals, each object alive with the spirit of the plants, animals, stones, and minerals with which it is made, and the thoughts, feelings, joy, and intent of the maker.

The Karuk kept the world harmonious through prayerful thoughts, actions, and offerings, adherence to rules of proper behavior, and the observance of spiritual dances in the proper season on a yearly cycle. A diverse set of "rules," both spiritual and practical, provided the underpinnings of the more commonplace aspects of day-to-day plant use, the most important and enduring to always give back for what is taken. The Karuk recited "formulas" when they gathered plants, including herbs.

> Herb doctors ... gather and then "talk to" the plants—that is, he or she recites a creation story, called a formula, over the herbs. Only then are they considered medicine. For us the healing spirit is not of the present. The spiritual power that invigorates the healing process is always ancient, and always from the creation times. The stories are essential to release the healing medicines of the earth. (Lang 1994: 30–31)

Even when the old-time formulas aren't known, Karuk plant gatherers, such as Kathy McCovey, seek to embody the spirit of those formulas in how they approach the plants:

> I don't know the formulas, or the prayers for individual plants, but when I go out, I always talk. ... It's like I'm talking to the plants, just like I'm talking to you. ... I really feel that the plant has energy, and it has a spirit just like me. (Personal communication with Beverly Ortiz, August 29, 1997)

Scores of non-Indian gold seekers invaded this thousands-of-years-old world of balance in 1850 to 1851. By some accounts, nearly 1,000 miners intruded, each one seeking their personal fortune. Although most had left by 1852, when the relatively easy to mine surface gold was gone, they left behind a legacy of incalculable tragedy—displacement, death and destruction, muddy rivers, and epidemics of consumption. The miners burned most Karuk villages as far north as the Salmon River, where Josephine Peters grew up. Hydraulic mining washed away others.

During this time, most Karuk were forced to flee into the mountains for safety. When they returned, non-Indian homes and farms had replaced their own homes and they were left to reestablish themselves where they could. Julian Lang has described the effect of the first half century of non-Indian intrusion as an "apocalypse" for his people. Wrote Lang in 1994: "The problems caused by the Forty-niners' thirst for gold at all costs, both human and environmental, are only now beginning to be resolved, one hundred and forty-four years later" (p. 11).

In 1908, Karuk country was still relatively isolated beyond Orleans Bar, with narrow foot and horse trails, often precarious and not well marked, following the river, far below, and river crossings made in redwood dugouts. A stage could not be accessed until reaching Forks of Salmon, some 24 miles distant, about 17 miles beyond Somes Bar. Somes Bar, located near the Three Dollar Bar ranch where Josephine Peters would be born fifteen years later, had a hotel, store, and barn in 1908, all later washed out in a flood. As described by Arnold and Reed (1957: 33): "Even on bright days, there are only three hours of sunshine in Somesbar [sic] in the wintertime. No one can cross the Salmon by dugout; the current runs too swift and the rocks are too dangerous." Instead, a swinging bridge had been constructed for crossing the racing river above a narrow gorge, with twelve-inch planks laid end to end and two steel cables (Arnold and Reed 1957: 27–41). Even with the building of paved roads and vehicle bridges, which occurred not long after Josephine was born, the area has retained its rugged beauty, although the rivers have been diminished because of distant water diversion projects (Most 2006), and the vegetation has become denser, due to the discontinuation of old-time land management practices.

FAMILY HISTORY

Because this is a very personal ethnobotany, rooted in the particular life history of Josephine Grant Peters, the details of Josephine's family history provide an essential backdrop for fuller appreciation of the grace, wisdom, and good nature with which Josephine has lived her life and the reasons that her plant knowledge is so multifaceted and dynamic. They root her to place and illuminate the reasons that she is genealogically and culturally Karuk, while she is also genealogically Konomihu/Shasta, Rouge River, and Abenaki. They explain the circumstances that led two individuals from opposite sides of the continent—one Abenaki from the east coast, the other Rogue River and Konomihu from the west coast—to meet and marry at such an early date, about 1852. Most importantly, they put a spotlight on the courage, resourcefulness, and resilience that enabled Josephine's ancestors to survive, and even thrive, despite the unfathomable upheaval, disruption, tragedy, cruelty, and sadness of the history that they lived through.

After describing the history of Josephine's paternal and maternal family, the focus of this chapter will shift to the details of Josephine's life. It will end with a description of a decades-long cultural revitalization in Karuk, Yurok, and Hupa country, the revitalization of which Josephine has been an important part.

In keeping with a personal focus of this ethnobotany, Josephine's own words have been interspersed throughout the text. You'll find these highlighted in italics.

Paternal Family History

Frank A. Grant III, Josephine's nephew, has traced the family's lineage back to 1759, with the birth of Francois Joseph Annance (Abenaki), who married Marie Josephete Thomas, also Abenaki. Three generations later, on November 28, 1827, Josephine's paternal great-grandfather, Francis (Frank) Brazille/Lagrave, was born in French Canada to Francis Brazille/Lagrave (born ca. 1803) and Ursule Wasaminet (Lucy Emmett, born ca. 1805), both Abenaki. Lagrave was the family's French Canadian name; Brazille their name in the United States.

When Francis, the younger, was a child, the Lagrave family lived at Saint Francis Indian Village (Odenak) in Quebec, where his father was an ash-splint basket maker. Their ancestors arrived at Saint Francis sometime in the 1700s as refugees of battles with English colonists in the United States. The Brazille/Lagrave family appears to be one of many Abenaki families who, in the 1800s, returned to their ancestral homeland in the United States to serve as hunters, guides, and participants in the ash-splint basketry tourist industry.

Francis Brazille, the oldest of eight full siblings, emigrated to northern California in 1849 as part of a gold rush–bound mining company. He began his cross-country journey in Sharon Springs, Schoharie County, New York, where his family had moved by 1845. In April 1849, the company camped in Saint Joseph, Missouri, awaiting the growth of grass tall enough to feed their animals on the trail (Grant III 2000: 1–4).

Census records show Francis living in Union Town (now Arcata in coastal northern California) in 1850. He appears to have met Isaac J. Wistar, a European American from Philadelphia, this same year. In Wistar's 1914 autobiography, he writes with great fondness about Francis and with great candor about their exploits. This rare, early account of an American Indian man by a non-Indian is notable for its humanity and detail and it will be quoted in part below. As Wistar remembered "Francois Bisell," he was "six feet high, handsome and well proportioned, fearless in character though extremely amiable, and was by far the best hunter I have ever met" (p. 197).

Wistar, born November 14, 1827, two weeks before Francis, had set off on a journey from Philadelphia to the gold fields on April 5, 1849. In his autobiography, Wistar described his eventual voyage from San Francisco to Trinidad, California, about 15 miles north of Arcata, to become a packer, ferrying supplies by burro, and later mules, to mining camps along the Klamath River. He first met Francis when the two men teamed up to kill a grizzly bear that had been depredating a store south of Trinidad (Wistar 1914: 42, 175–187).

In subsequent weeks, the two men traveled and camped together, at one point confronting, at gunpoint, some non-Indians about to execute three Indians who were falsely accused of killing cattle near Trinidad.

> We had been up the coast some miles above Trinidad to an Indian village where we occasionally got a sea otter skin or two, and were returning to camp by way of Trinidad, the only available mule trail lying through the town. On emerging from the "one mile gulch" just above the town, we came upon several of the boiled-shirt gentry (gamblers) who had three Indians bound to trees

and were discussing in what manner to put them to death. The Indians, who knew us, called on us to save them, and we recognized them as inhabitants of the village we had just come from. Some cattle had been killed near the town, and the gamblers, who knew nothing of Indians … had seized these poor friendlies who were in frequent and amicable communication with packers and fur men. …

… F. possessed that dangerous sort of temperament [sic] that becomes cooler in exact proportion as danger comes nearer, and at the very crisis, he was sure to be almost painfully deliberate. Without taking his eyes an instant from the enemy, he remarked to me in a drawling tone in Chinook "Will you fight?" "Yes." … Suddenly drawing his rifle F. ordered "Throw down your pistols. Hands up!"

… They were well huddled up together, and may have had time to reflect that at their first hostile motion two or more would be dead for certain, with a smart chance for some more. At any rate, the order was obeyed and their pistols assured. (Wistar 1914: 197–199)

These non-Indian gamblers apparently controlled the town, and soon Francis and Wistar teamed up with eleven other "mountain men" to undertake a surprise raid on the Trinidad gambling house where the gamblers resided. After separating and fleeing the area, Francis and Wistar met again. Broke, despising the "regular humdrum labor of mining," and with their raid on the gambling house still fresh, they determined to head for the Columbia, where Francis had been a trapper for the Hudson Bay Company (Wistar 1914: 200–206). According to Wistar, Francis,

was as experienced a trapper, hunter and traveler, as was to be found throughout all its vast territory. There was no fish, bird or animal whose habits and resorts he did not know. If there was a deer anywhere within ten miles he was sure to find it, and I doubt whether he had a superior anywhere as a mountain man and hunter. I never knew him to lose his bearings in the most intricate and perplexing mountain ranges, except on a few occasions in consequence of my bad advice, and then, when I gave it up, he was always able to rectify it quickly, and I never heard a reproach from his lips. (Wistar 1914: 208)

The two men made their way by horseback "into the Rocky Mountains by the Smoky Fork of the Peace." Their late arrival coincided with a lack of either marten or game (Wistar 1914: 206–213), and Wistar wrote forcefully about how Francis's knowledge, skill, calm disposition, flexibility, and faith saved them from near starvation.

After trying in vain all the resources practised [sic] by trappers in such straits, all of which were well known to Francois, we ate the grease in our rifle stocks, all the fringes and unnecessary parts of our buck leather clothes, gun and ammunition bags, and every scrap of eatable material, boiling it down in an Assinaboine basket with hot stones, and were finally reduced to buds and twigs. … At this last stage in the struggle, an event occurred of the most extraordinary character. … Notwithstanding our exhaustion … F. rose at daylight, made up the fire as well as his strength permitted, blazed a tree near by [sic] on which he marked with charcoal a large cross, and carefully reloading and standing his gun against that emblem, proceeded to repeat in such feeble whispers as he was yet capable of, all the scraps of French and Latin prayers he could remember. … [S]carcely a few minutes had elapsed, and as it afterwards appeared he had hardly traversed a couple of hundred yards, when I heard his gun, which I knew never cracked in vain. ...

... Two good hunters had ransacked the vicinity for miles without finding a living thing, and had tried in vain all the numerous resources known to the trapper, when a caribou, the wildest and most timid of all deer, walks right into camp, as one may say, at the last moment when further delay was death. ... Francois believed, and till his latest breath will continue to believe, that after all human efforts had been put forth in vain, the holy Saint Francis, his patron saint, moved by his suffering and prayer, had himself bared an arm for our relief. (Wistar 1914: 214–215)

Eventually, the two men separated, and by 1852 Francis had become a resident of Klamath, now Siskiyou County, in northern California, where he married Queen. Queen's grandmother, who was raised in Yreka, married a Rouge River Indian, who brought her to his southern Oregon homeland, where they raised a large family. Massacres of Indians by non-Indians had become commonplace by the time Queen's mother was born, and she fled, as a grown woman, from Oregon to Salmon River country. Once there, she married a Konomihu, one of the Shasta tribes. Their daughter Queen was born in the 1830s, in the vicinity of Scott Valley, in Shasta tribal territory (see Figure 1.2) (Grant III 1972: 15, III 2000: 12; Wistar 1914: 2).

The Brazille family established a cattle ranch and farm, with "abundant quantities of fine fruit and vegetables," and a mining operation, at Forks of Salmon, where the North and South Forks of the Salmon River meet, about sixteen miles downriver of Somes Bar, near Three Dollar Bar, the place where Josephine would be born seventy-one years later. As an American Indian, Francis could not legally own land, so to obtain his ranch, he identified himself as French (Grant III 2000: 1–2, 6, 11).

Some twenty-six or so years after he established himself at Forks of Salmon, Francis, whose courage had sustained him as a youth, died on January 18, 1878, of lingering complications from being struck on the head with a pick handle during a fight the previous June. After his death, Queen continued to live on the Forks of Salmon property with some of her children, until she died in the 1890s (Grant III 1972: 15, 2000: 11).

Josephine's grandmother Ellen Brazille, the second daughter of Francis and Queen Brazille, was born about 1856 (Grant III 1972: 15). She was brought by Francis and Queen to the village known as Wahp-sah-kah-ahch-te-ah, or Inskips, when she was a young child. There she was raised among the Konomihu, in whose language she became fluent. In 1921, Ellen served as cultural consultant for anthropologist C. Hart Merriam. Through Merriam, we get a small window into some of the qualities that both Ellen and her granddaughter Josephine share—a keen intellect and remarkable memory (see Figure 1.3) (Heizer 1967: 230).[4]

Ellen Brazille married Hugh Grant, who was born ca. 1847 in Nova Scotia, Canada. After emigrating west as a young man, he worked as a "chopper" in the vicinity of Arcata before making his way to the Salmon River to mine gold (Grant III 1972: 15). Josephine had this to say about her grandfather in 1998:

I remember that my grandpa died when I was only three years old, but I remember him, and I can remember his hands, he had real big hands, and he was a miner that came from Nova Scotia. He mined along the Salmon River. They had a homestead that was called Butler Flats, and he mined across the river, and he mined the upper part of the property. (Marshall 1998: 9).

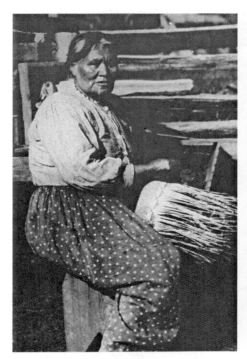

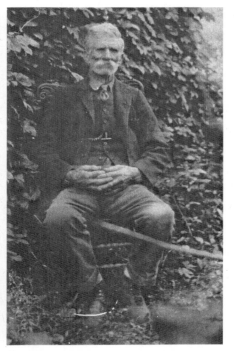

Figure 1.2. *(Left)* Josephine's paternal great-grandmother Queen Brazille weaving a basket. Photo courtesy Josephine Peters.

Figure 1.3. *(Right)* Josephine's paternal grandfather Hugh Grant. Photo courtesy Josephine Peters.

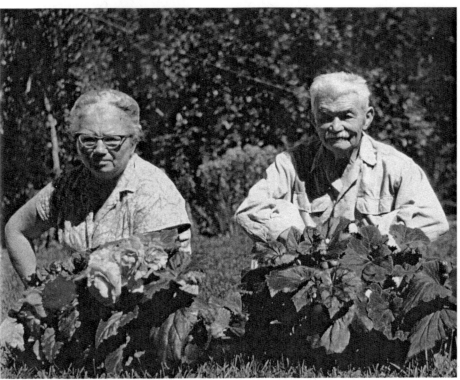

Figure 1.4. Josephine's parents Maggie Bennett Grant and Frank A. Grant with their begonias at the Old Home Place, where Josephine was born, near Somes Bar. Photo courtesy Josephine Grant Peters.

At Butler Flat, Hugh and Ellen raised nine children, two of whom died young. Josephine's father Frank A. Grant, their fifth child, was born April 22, 1888 (see Figure 1.4) (Frank Grant III 1972: 15–16, 19).

Figure 1.5.
Josephine Peters and daughter
Cheryl at the Old Home Place,
with Josephine's mother Maggie
Bennett holding Cheryl's daugh-
ter Colette, 1963. Photo courtesy
Josephine Peters.

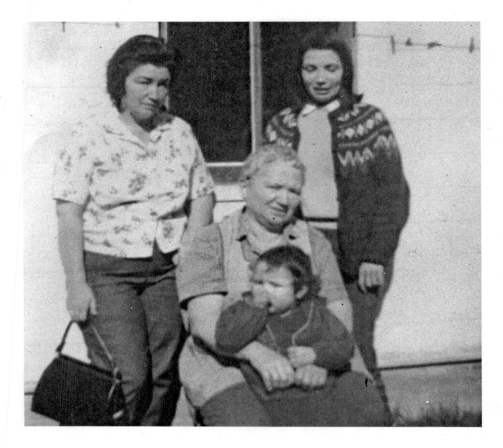

Maternal Family History

Josephine's mother Maggie Bennett was born May 24, 1902, to George Bennett (1877–1934) and Louise Nelson (1881–1966). George Bennett's father was William Porter Bennett, born 1832, in Sangamon County, Illinois. William Porter Bennett arrived in Shasta County, California, in 1853, after crossing the plains with, it appears, his uncle Robert Bennett and other friends. He soon took up gold mining in Trinity County, engaging in "Indian skirmishes in the winter of 1854–55." In 1856, William Porter Bennett relocated on the forks of the Salmon River, where he mined, had a trading post, and ran a pack train. He entered the merchandising business in Cecilville with the purchase of the P.F. Dunphy store. In 1873, he established himself at Forks of Salmon, where he purchased another store and had a stable, hotel, and stage station (see Figure 1.5).

William Porter Bennett married Sarah Crawford (1837–1882) at Orleans on September 26, 1869. They had five children, including George. Two years later, William Porter Bennett married Melissa L. Crawford (1850–1914), who came to California in 1869.

When William Porter Bennett first came to the area he lived with Julie Miller (Karuk). They had a son, John, who was also married to Louise Nelson, Scandinavian on her father Hans Nelson's side, and Karuk and Shasta on her mother Jennie Redcap Johnnie 's side. Jennie Johnnie later married Redcap Johnnie, after Hans Nelson disappeared (see Figure 1.6) (Grant III 1972: 19; Cheryl Beck, personal communication with Beverly Ortiz, September 27, 2009).

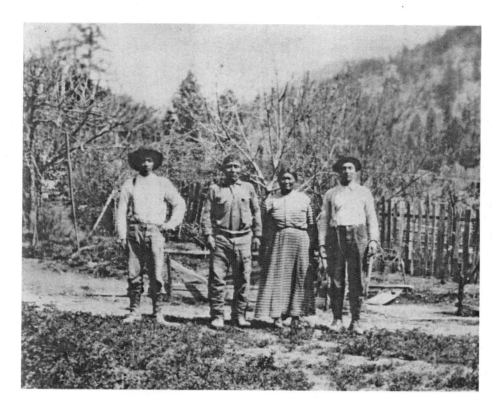

Figure 1.6.
Unidentified man, Redcap Johnnie, Jennie Redcap Johnnie, and
Peters Thomas, who married
one of the sisters of Josephine's
mother Maggie Bennett. Photo
courtesy Josephine Peters.

JOSEPHINE GRANT PETERS

Childhood

Josephine Peters was born on March 8, 1923, near Somes Bar, California, the second of the eleven children of Frank A. Grant, Sr. (Nova Scotian/Karuk/Konhomini/ Rouge River/Abenaki), and Maggie Bennett (Karuk/Shasta/Scandinavian): Frank Jr., Josephine, Reginald, Beryl, Vivienna, Wayne, Byron, Delbert, Melissa, Mildred, and Maurice. Josephine and her siblings grew up at Three Dollar Bar along the Salmon River, her school a six-mile round trip walk. In the wintertime, the children left for Junction School in the dark; they also returned in the dark. *Sometimes there'd be three or four feet of snow. My dad used to lead a horse through to break trail, and we'd walk* (see Figure 1.7 and Figure 1.8).

Before heading off to school, Josephine and her siblings rose before daybreak to complete a variety of chores. These included feeding the horses, feeding and milking the cows, and tending the chickens. During haying season, they raked the hay into mounds and loaded it on the wagon. When Josephine started school, one room served all eight grades. By the time she graduated, a second room had been added, and a second teacher, Minerva Staritt.

The Grant family was largely self-sufficient, with garden, fruit trees, cattle, and hay. "*Old mutts*" helped with the hunting, treeing bears, and raccoons—the bear fat was rendered for grease; the raccoons were cooked for chicken feed. Frank Grant, a skilled carpenter, mason, rancher, logger, and sometimes miner, was often away from home. His children participated in a bit of his mining activities, however, particularly the annual assessment work.

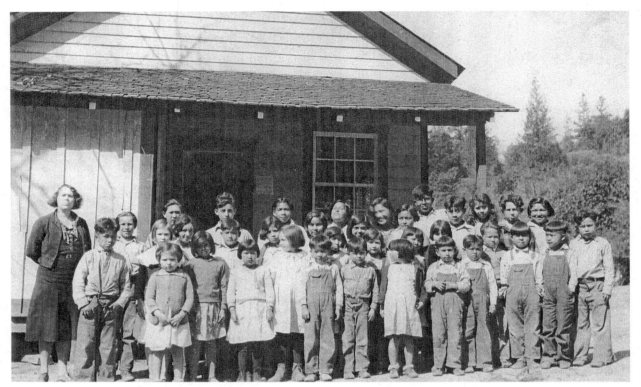

Figure 1.7.
1933–1934 Junction School class, Somes Bar, taken when Josephine was in the sixth grade. Photo courtesy Zona Ferris, who identified the children in the photograph. Originally published in Graves (1934). *Front row, left to right*: Frederick Case (?), Loretta McNeil, Lorella Conrad, Goldie Tom, Anna McNeil, Wilfred Albers, Ernest Conrad, Margie Johnson (?), Art Case, Arnold Davis, Frederick Case (?), Loren Offield, Alfred Albers. *Second row, left to right*: Elsa M. Williams, Howard Shinski, Zona Ferris, Josephine Peters, Leland Donahue, Fern Grant, Maryanne Albers, Beverly Donahue (between Wilfred and Ernest), Ethel Drake Ferris (between Ernest and Margie), two unidentified girls (behind Margie and Art), Dorothy Albers (?) and Anabel, Reginald "Reggie" Grant. *Back row, left to right*: Lee Merrill (between Zona and Josephine), Frank Grant (behind Leland), Shane Davis (behind Fern), Vardina Donahue, Pauline Conrad (between Beverly and Ethel), Rosie Jerry Grant (slightly out of focus), Caroline Davis Brown, Wilson Donahue (slightly behind Caroline), Julius Tripp, Barbara Grant, Tommy Offield (?), Violet Johnny Super.

Every year you had to do so much digging on your property. He used to tell us to dig a big hole and an assessment would be marked so many yards. It had to be done every year if you had a mining camp. (Marshall 1998: 9–10)

After high waters, Josephine would sometimes pull nuggets from a particular rock: *I found some nuggets, we used to stay at the high waters and go up the big rock. We would put a stick in the big rock and use tweezers to pull* [the gold] *out.* Sluice boxes provided one method to separate the gold from riverine sands and gravel. Quicksilver (mercury) allowed the gold to collect in a lump, then Josephine and her older siblings would pan it out as it came through the boxes (Marshall 1998:10).

There was hydraulic mining, and then my dad made us a rocker. ... [W]e would put our gravel into this screen box and shake it back and forth and all of the sand and gold would go through, and the rocks, we would throw off to the side. So that was easier than panning, we could work through a lot of gravel that way. (Marshall 1998: 10).

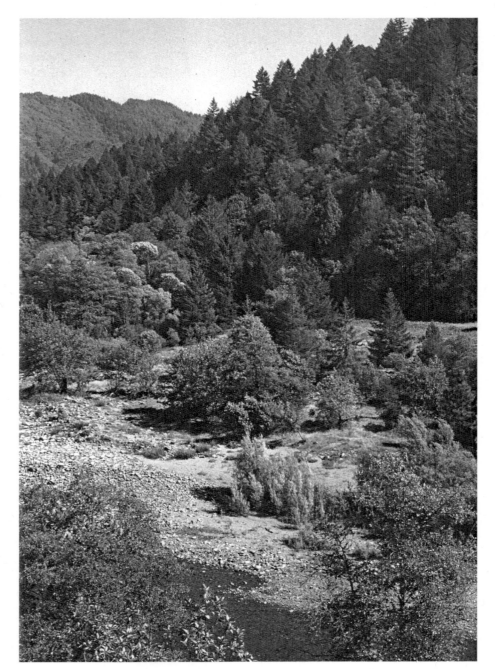

Figure 1.8.
Landscape at the Old Home
Place. Photo by Beverly Ortiz,
August 30, 2001.

Josephine's uncle and aunt Carl and Melissa Langford operated a store below their
Somes Bar home. The children climbed a nearby fig tree, whenever they craved one of
its fruits. Until Josephine was six, when her first sister was born, she had only boys to
play with—five brothers and young uncles. Josephine relished playing the boy's com-
petitive games, including competitions to see who could eat the most garlic. Josephine
thought nothing of wrestling with the boys: *We used to wrassle like heck for a quarter
or a dime*, Josephine explained with a laugh. Running up hills and hiding behind trees
during games of tag also provided hours of entertainment (see Figure 1.9).

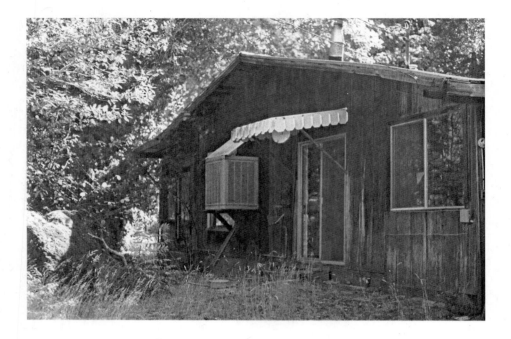

Creativity and imagination were the order of the day, as Josephine and the boys fashioned objects from clay: *And one time* [laughs] *when my mother was gone, my older brother and I made mud pies, and I sneaked some sugar and put it in ...* [laughs] *My brother says it's the best mud pie he ever ate!* [laughs]

A large, bush-like peppernut near home, where quail congregated, provided a special retreat. Dare-devil activities included swinging from limb to limb in the biggest, tallest, oldest pepperwood [bay] trees, breaking limbs and falls taken in stride: *Every time my folks were gone, we tried something. ... Soon as they were gone, we'd go get our pole and start pole vaulting up to the top of the house. We used to go down to the barn and walk the poles across the top of the hay. ... We tried everything.* [laughs] An old donkey was fun to ride. When the donkey had enough, it would run under an apple tree and scrape the children off.

The Somes Bar covered bridge, which washed out in the 1955 flood, provided an unusual source of diversion during Josephine's grammar school years in the late 1920s and early 1930s. The children would climb underneath it. From the inside they made their voices echo. Barrels on either end of the bridge held water in case a fire erupted. The children dipped cans into that water then threw it at each other.

At school, the children slid down the nearby serpentine hillside on homemade sleds, dodging the large oak in their path. To make their sleds, the children looked for a tree with a bend, cut it down, and whittled it into runner. Then they nailed boards across (see Figure 1.10).

During the summer, Josephine and her siblings spent time living with their paternal Aunt Ida, whose husband worked for the Forest Service. Aunt Ida taught Josephine to make rag dolls, take socks with red heels and turn them into red-nosed monkeys, and make quilts.

Josephine began learning basketry as a child from Phoebe Maddux (Karuk), who lived about three-quarters of a mile away, and her maternal great-aunts, Minnie Ruben Johnnie (Karuk) and Mary Johnnie (Karuk), with and for whom she gathered

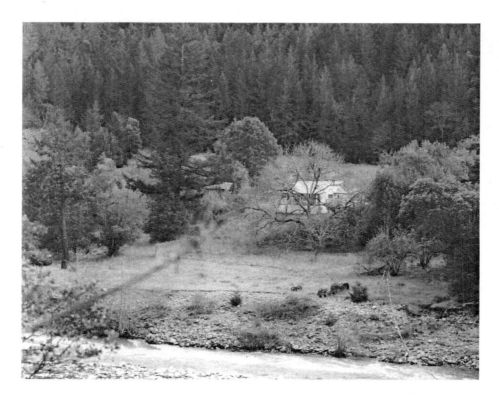

Figure 1.10.
Old Home Place with barn visible in distance. Photo by George Beck, courtesy of Cheryl Beck.

"sticks" for their baskets. Josephine started learning the weaving process by trial and error, when she was about eight or nine years old, based on what she observed (Johnson and Marks 1997: 128).

> *I used to sit out in the yard with picked plantain, those big high stems and weave with that. But we had a fire one time, up right above our house, a ways, that burned the mountain off; so the next spring this old lady and I went out. She came early in the morning with her lunch and wood basket. We went up there and picked hazel sticks all day on the side of the hill.... We took a load down, ... and then we ate our lunch, then* [we] *went back up and down. I thought she was going to say, "Let's go home."* [We] *went back up again ... and we really had a load to pack coming out of there.* (Johnson and Marks 1997: 128)

Minnie Johnnie was known for her miniatures. Mary Johnnie lived along Josephine's route to and from school.

> *I'd leave school and go over to stay at her place and sit on her porch and watch her make baskets. Then she'd tell me how. She showed me how to make those knots ... to hold the baby baskets and plate baskets together. ... I'd sit there and practice making* [those] *knots.* (Johnson and Marks 1997: 128)

Mary taught Josephine to make open-work baskets; Phoebe Maddox showed her how to start the closed-twined ones. When she was young, Josephine specialized in the making of handle, baby, and clothes baskets with hazel, as well as finely woven hats and gift baskets. After a stroke at age 23, she could no longer make the full-size utilitarian baskets but continued to exercise her hands by quilting and crocheting afghans. She eventually resumed making closed-twined baskets.

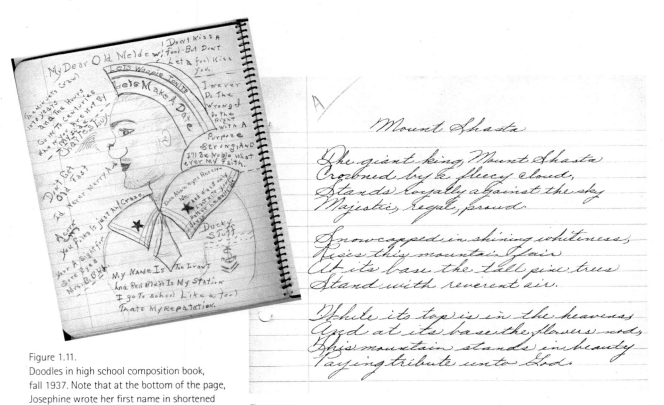

Figure 1.11.
Doodles in high school composition book, fall 1937. Note that at the bottom of the page, Josephine wrote her first name in shortened form as "Joe," although later in life she preferred "Jo." Courtesy Josephine Peters.

Figure 1.12.
Mount Shasta poem composed by Josephine for high school English II class, 1939. Courtesy of Josephine Peters.

When Josephine graduated from grammar school, Mary Johnny wove a basket cap for her with the family design on it, triangular people sitting around a larger, triangular fire. Josephine graduated with two other students, Zona Ferris and Glen Gallop. According to Zona Ferris, their class motto was: "The cutest class this side of heaven. The class of 1937" (personal communication with Beverly Ortiz, July 2005; see Figure 1.11 and Figure 1.12).

After graduation, Josephine moved to Red Bluff, where she attended ninth grade while living with her maternal great-aunt Millie. In 1938, she returned home for a year, then moved to Etna to resume her education. When Josephine graduated from high school in Etna in 1942, her great-aunt made her a second basket cap. That year she moved to Eureka, where, when World War II broke out, she worked as a welder in a shipyard dry dock. She stayed a year and a half before moving to Arcata to care for the baby of a young mother who died in childbirth. When the war ended, Josephine returned to Eureka before moving to Ford Ord, where she folded bandages. Next, she relocated to Palm Springs to be near her uncle, who was in an army hospital being treated for severe injuries he received during a war-time explosion. While there, Josephine cared for patients with leg injuries.

Josephine returned briefly to Eureka, then moved to Trinidad for a few years. She stayed there until 1949, when she came to Hoopa, where she has resided ever since.

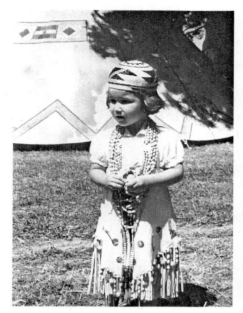

Figure 1.13.
Tamara Peters in dance regalia made by her mother.
Ella Johnson likely made the cap. Humboldt County
Fair, Ferndale. Photo courtesy Josephine Peters.

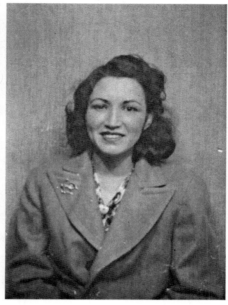

Figure 1.14.
Josephine Peters in the 1950s. Photo courtesy Josephine Peters.

Motherhood

Place, culture, extended family, and community have been interconnected constants throughout Josephine's life, as they have been for her people across millennia. At once self-sufficient yet also part of an interdependent system of daily interactions—with people and with the landscape—the values of giving, caring, and sharing have suffused Josephine's life.

Josephine's daughter Cheryl Gerchia Beck was born in 1943. Cheryl's father Thomas Gerchia (Garcia) died in World War II. Daughter Tamara C. Peters was born in 1963, three weeks after her father Charles "Slim" Peters died in a logging accident (see Figure 1.13).

In 1949, living in Hoopa, Josephine began taking in foster children, twenty-seven in all. She served as guardian for as many as five children at a time, until her large home was destroyed in the 1964 flood. Fortunately, there was enough warning of the impending flood that Josephine was able to save her baskets, other cultural objects, and memorabilia, but not the furnishings (see Figure 1.14).

On October 28, 1980, Josephine adopted Quetta Peters (Cree). In 1992, she decided to become the guardian of Jene McCovey, whom she took in as a baby: *I was getting old. It was time to retire. I turned around and got another one. ... I started all over again* [laughs].

As a mother, Josephine emphasized the importance of education and good employment. She delighted in each child's graduation and reveled in each professional accomplishment. Quetta Peters' 2004 reflections about her mother provide insight about Josephine's influence on all her children (see Figure 1.15).

Most people who have been fortunate enough to sit and talk with her know the inner strength and wisdom she possesses. She's a person who sees past what most people generally see, deep into one's own soul. Her kindness and generosity are abundant. She would give the shirt off her own back to another human being if they needed it more than her.

My mother has more cultural knowledge about plants, basketry, arts and crafts, language and religion, as well as "general native psychology," than any other person I know. She unselfishly shares her knowledge with others, teaching basketry, for instance, for more years than I've even been alive. She continues to be a role model for many young people. Her presence at most culturally-related functions is a blessing. For example, in a few days she will attend a graduation gathering of the Tribal Civilian Community Corps in Hoopa to wish the graduates of the program well and to send "Good Medicine" their way.

My mom taught us the vital importance of maintaining good health, preparing three well-balanced meals throughout my childhood. I might not have always liked the veggie part, but there's lots of love in her traditional home cooking. She taught me to prepare acorn soup (I think hers is superb!), as well as eels, salmon, and deer and elk meat, just to name a few. I am a skilled cook because of my mother. (Personal communication with Beverly Ortiz, May 11, 2004)

In 2004, Cheryl Beck's granddaughter Samantha "Sam" McDonald, who lives out-of-state, aptly described her great-grandmother's influence on her (see Figure 1.16):

My great-grandma Jo, to me, is just plain and amazing. … I lived with her in Hoopa during the summers of 2002 and 2003. I got to really know my Grandma Jo then. For the very first time I could actually talk to her like an adult. I could carry on a conversation with her, which I couldn't do before. I was now a teenager, and people finally took me seriously.

The first summer I stayed with Grandma Jo was after seventh grade. Her daughter, my Grandma Beck, my sister Rebecca, and Grandma Jo all went down to the CIBA (California Indian Basketweavers Association) convention. This experience really opened my eyes to my culture. I watched my Grandma Jo help my big sister weave a basket, and I just wished so badly that I could weave like my family. My chance came. My Great-Grandma Jo and Grandma Beck both helped me to pick out a class. They picked out classes they thought would interest me, and I chose the Karuk fishtrap basket class. One of my cousins was teaching that particular class, and once I got started my Grandma Jo helped me by showing me what to do and what mistakes I had made. As soon as I finished one basket, my Great-Grandma Jo started me on another basket, and I have been working on that one.

While I was at the CIBA convention, I saw a tribal dance, and I wished that I could have danced. I wanted to dance so much that I told my sister, and she said I probably could learn. My Great-Grandma Jo heard us talking and began to tell me about my Karuk tribal dances, which made me want to learn even more. Grandma Jo started giving me directions on what to do, how to stand, and the behavior of girl dancers, plus other things.

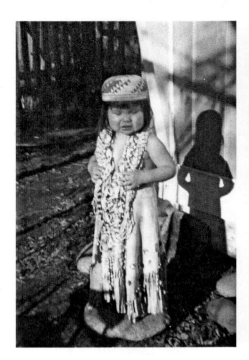 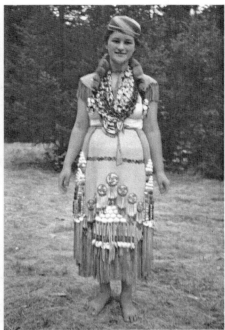

Figure 1.15. *(Left)* Quetta Peters at home wearing regalia made by Josephine. Basket hat with rivers and mountain design likely made by Ella Johnson. Photo courtesy Josephine Peters.

Figure 1.16. *(Right)* Josephine's great-granddaughter Samantha McDonald in regalia and basket hat with whirlwind design, all made by Josephine. Photo by Beverly Ortiz.

I asked her when the next dance would be held, and she told me the next Brush Dance would be held that coming weekend. Then I asked her if I could stay in Hoopa for part of the summer to dance. She told me it would be fine, but that I had to ask my Mom and Grandma Beck first. They all agreed, so I got to stay, and that weekend I got to dance in a Brush Dance for the very first time, and I was almost jumping for joy, but at the same time a little scared. I danced and people, including my Great-Grandma Jo, told me they were proud of me, and that I was doing good things for my family as well. I danced a few more times while I was in Hoopa that summer, and I loved every moment of it.

When I look at all the Indian dresses, the basket caps and regalia that my Great-Grandma Jo has or has made, I would dream of making a dress or regalia of my own. I made a few things, and I have been trying, but nothing will be anything like my Great-Grandma Jo's.

All in all I had fun that summer, and I loved everything I saw and did. Looking at my Great-Grandma Jo's dresses just amazed me; the fact that she had made several of those dresses just made me go, "Wow!"

The summers I spent with Great-Grandma Jo, she taught me so much, almost by accident. She would show me an herb and tell me what it could be used for, and when and how to harvest it. I would just pick stuff up. Now it is at the point where people ask me who I am related to, and when I tell them, they know exactly who I am talking about, and it is sort of an honor to introduce myself as the Great-Granddaughter of Jo Peters. I don't think it can get much better than that. There are three women in my life that I really respect with all my heart. They are my Mom, my Grandma Beck and my Great-Grandma Jo. (Personal communication with Cheryl Beck, March 2004)

Becoming an Herbalist

Anybody's welcome if they want to learn. [...] [One] Indian doctor doesn't want me to do this. She said, "You're giving our secrets." I told her, "Somebody's got to know." (Josephine Peters, July 15, 1998)

Josephine's herbalism rests on the firmest of foundations—family legacy.[5] Her paternal great-grandmother Queen Brazille was an Indian doctor. In 1928, Susan Brazille, Josephine's paternal great-aunt, explained the genesis of Queen's herbal knowledge to linguist J. P. Harrington (Mills 1985: II/30, 38).

Susan's maternal grandfather was a doctor. He taught Susan many herbs. Used to be lots of Spanish around here. The Spanish and whites called him Mawima. That (is his Indian?) name. When he died he gave his doctorship to Colonel, his son (Susan's uncle), and when Colonel died he gave the knowledge of herbs to Queen, Susan's mother. Whites used to call her Queen, for she was a pretty-looking woman. Whites when they got sick used to go to Mawima to be treated. (Grant III 2000: 12)

Queen's daughter, Josephine's paternal-grandmother Ellen Brazille, continued her mother's legacy, and prepared many herbal remedies for her grandchildren. In retrospect, Josephine thinks that a lot of these remedies may have been brewed from St. John's wort, an herb that settles the stomach. *If we got sick, she'd mix up something for us to take. Those days, we never knew what she was giving us.*

Josephine has always had a propensity for learning about herbs. She has many fond childhood memories of the times she spent following various older, local women around, wherever they went, noticing what they picked, and asking questions about the plants. *I'd be like Jene.* [laughs] *I'd ask questions until I found out what they were using it for... Different elderly ladies would say, "Well this is good for that. That's good for that." They were midwives. Every time they had to go, they'd send me: "Hurry up. Run down. Dig that up."*

When it came to certain plants, like Solomon seal, the women instilled an enduring sense of cautious respect: *[T]hey used to tell us, "Don't touch it; it's poison," when we used to walk by it. Then when they needed it, they'd send us to get it. It was a narcotic. ... That's why they didn't want us to bother it.*

From the women, she also learned that an important aspect of interacting with plants included talking to them before gathering, letting them know, for instance, "I'm picking this herb to use for medicine." Sometimes, she advises, a song will come during gathering, a song that leaves you when you leave the gathering area.[6]

When Josephine attended junior high school in Red Bluff during the 1937–38 school year, her classmates included two sons of a Chinese herbalist, Mr. Yen. She joined the brothers in gathering herbs for their father, incorporating some of them into her repertoire of herbal remedies, including lady slipper and knotweed.

At age twenty-three, Josephine had her first stroke, and she knew it was time to renew her family's doctoring legacy.[7] Initially, she only used herbal medicines on herself. Within about two years, she had started to prescribe them to others.

As word about the effectiveness of Josephine's herbal remedies spread, she began to receive invitations to share her knowledge with a wider audience, including students at Humboldt State University and the University of California, Riverside. In the 1970s and '80s, she was invited to doctoring conferences, where she had an opportunity to compare her herbal remedies with that of other Indian herbalists and

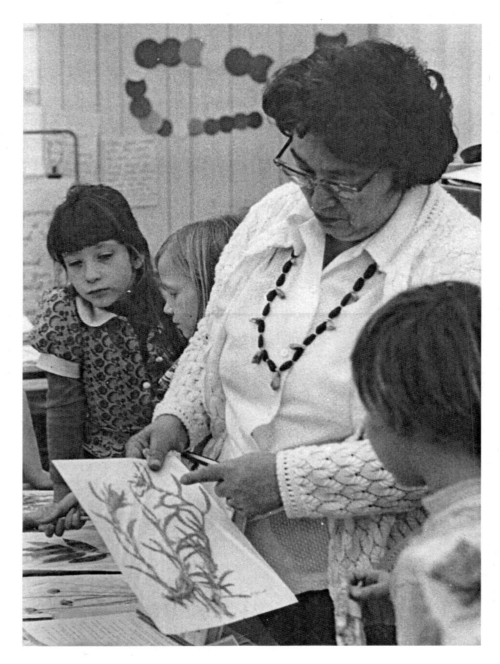

Figure 1.17.
Josephine, wearing a necklace she made, sharing the uses of a pressed herbs with school children. Photo courtesy Josephine Peters.

doctors. This included three visits to South America to study with herbalists there. *I've gone to Canada a couple of times on it. And then I went to Bogotá. We stayed at the University of Bogotá. ... Then I went to Peru. That was interesting, because we got to go ... up to Machu Picchu.*

Closer to home, Josephine was an active participant in Hoopa Valley's Traditional Medicine Program, coordinated by Dr. Richard Ricklefs, who advised and assisted a community-wide effort to raise funds to build the Hoopa Medical Center in 1960, and who built a clinic near that hospital in 1962. The program's weekly meetings were designed to promote "holistic values in theory and diagnosis [that] make up traditional designs for treatment of health problems." These included guest speakers, among them local elders, Indian doctors from other areas, and a neurologist. The program focused on education about preventative medicine, and included the establishment of a library about holistic medicine, and the creation of "a register for cataloguing and dispensing herbs" (Common Sense 1980a: 10, 1980b:14, 1980c: 11, 12; Small 1980: 10): "In an effort to build up a register … , Everett Smith and Dr. Ricklefs along with Josephine Peters have been organizing field trips and have been conducting seminars on herbs and their uses" (Small 1980:10).

Josephine also had opportunities to share her knowledge of plant use at Chawse (Indian Grinding State Park) near Volcano, California, with participants in the annual gathering of the Committee for Traditional Indian Health, which was established in 1981. This program of the California Rural Indian Health Board is designed to inspire those present to "begin to seek knowledge of their tribe's medicines and cures" (Navarro 2000/01) (see Figure 1.17 on previous page).

Josephine also met with several Indian doctors who visited Hoopa Valley. She also corresponded with Indian doctors, exchanging herbs by mail. When learning about other doctors' plant uses, she found it easiest to remember those pertaining to plants that grew in her home country. Some plants prominent in other geographical areas also made a lasting impression, for example, oregano and devil's club.

> *There was this Indian doctor from Mexico. They believe in oregano. They use oregano for everything. Going up the coast into Alaska and British Columbia, it's all devil's club. … It grows from Orick north… [T]he natives up in Alaska cut it up and dry it. It's their big medicine up there. … I used to give it down here, but … not much. Only on poulticing.*

Josephine finds particular satisfaction in sharing her plant knowledge with doctors trained in modern medicine, so that they know what to prescribe when modern techniques don't offer a cure. Asked by individuals if she'll accept pay in exchange for the opportunity to study with her, Josephine responds emphatically: *I don't take money. … If you take money, you lose your power.*

The effectiveness of one of Josephine's poultices, and one of her salves, was put to the test in 2005, when eighth-grader Carlyn Girard decided to conduct an experiment for that year's California State Science Fair that would compare how well Karuk antibiotics and over-the-counter Neosporin killed the bacteria that cause skin infections. When Carlyn visited Humboldt State University to research Karuk antibiotics, so she could run her experiment, she was redirected to Josephine. To help Carlyn with the experiment, Josephine decided to prepare a pepperwood nutmeat leaf and olive oil poultice and a coltsfoot salve. Carlyn compared the effectiveness of these against two pure strains of bacteria (*Staphylococcus epidermis* and *Pseudomonas fluorescens*), and four wild strains of bacteria, that she harvested from her own skin. As Carlyn soon found out, the peppernut poultice and coltsfoot salve both had "significant antibacterial effects on common skin bacteria," with the peppernut poultice showing a larger no-growth zone than Neosporin against *Staphylococcus epidermis* bacteria. Coltsfoot was "effective" against *Bacillis subtilis* and *Streptobacillis bacteria*. In her project abstract Carlyn concluded: "Many bacteria that cause infections are showing more and more resistance to our modern antibiotics. My results show that these traditional Native American medicines may be a source of new antibacterial medicine" (www.usc.edu/CSSF/Current/Panels/J13. html). As a result of her experiment, Carlyn earned first place in the 2005 State

Science Fair's microbiology category, in competition with forty-one other statewide finalists in that category (Arthurs 2005).

Although Josephine has received much public recognition for her plant knowledge, she finds particular joy in sharing that knowledge one-on-one with community members. In 2005, Patricia Ferris (Hupa) recounted one memorable day when she had an opportunity to gather plants with Josephine:

> It was a couple of years ago in the fall of the year. It was a very special time in our lives. Our granddaughter Pateisha was having a Flower Dance in Hoopa. Everyone in the family had things to do or gather and not much time.
>
> I called Josephine to see if she would ride up with me to gather ginger. We went up to the spring and picked it. It was so beautiful that day, and both of us being mountain women, we decided to keep driving on up the mountain. We gathered cedar and white fir tips. We found a good place to pull off with a nice view of the mountains. We talked and told stories, and it turned out to be a wonderful day. I hope that we can get together again soon to enjoy the mountains and share stories about that dance and the up-river Jump Dance training Pateisha is getting now. (Personal communication, with Beverly Ortiz July 13, 2005)

A CULTURAL RENAISSANCE

Josephine grew up in an era of transition, when the practice of cultural traditions, such as basketry and ceremonies, was in decline.

> *After the whites came in here, they tried to rule all of us—tell us what to do, and take things away from us, like weaving baskets. When we saw somebody coming, we'd hide it; just grab everything up, and throw it behind a chair, or some other place, and cover it up with a towel. ... Well, after the government schools closed down, and everybody came back, most of the younger people had to learn the Indian ways all over again. A lot of them never did go back to it. ... Baskets were really dying out. Hardly anybody was making them anymore, because they had no [market] for it. They were scared to go out and sell it to someone, so we started making pottery.*

Hoopa Pottery Guild

The Hoopa Pottery Guild started in 1951 when Laura Black, a field nurse, noticed sources of clay on her journeys to Hoopa. After Black introduced the pottery-making process, Josephine became one of its most skilled and versatile artisans. Josephine completed her first pot in March 1953, a rusty-brown bowl with a pumpkin-orange mountain and river design outlined in black. Pinched from a ball of clay, it stands about two inches high and three inches across, a solid, triangular peak with ridges enveloping a zigzag river.

While local tribal peoples used baskets for all of their containers in the old days, basketry materials had become increasingly hard to obtain, and fewer and fewer women wove. According to Vivien Hailstone (Karuk/Yurok/Member of the Hoopa Tribe), as quoted in a 1967 newspaper article, pottery filled the void.

The designs and shapes of the pottery blend themselves well with the nearly lost native Indian art of basket weaving. ... Clay for the pottery is relatively easy to obtain. It can be found almost anywhere locally, and requires very little preparation. It does give us an outlet for expression of our native art. (Peters 1950s–1970s)

As guild membership grew, a pottery studio was built in Hoopa. Although the building was lost in the 1964 flood, in collaboration with community members, another was constructed in Hoopa on the Presbyterian Church grounds by Presbyterian youth from as far away as Hayward under the supervision of Reverend Charles Messinger, who "was also instrumental in raising money for the project" (Peters 1950s–1970s). The church eventually decided to discontinue the building's use for pottery making, but by that time individual members had acquired their own wheels and kilns, and continued their work at home.

Throughout the early years, when the guild members gathered, they discussed cultural traditions. Pride grew, and they eventually determined to begin teaching basketry. According to Josephine,

> *We tried to save the basket designs by putting it on pottery. And then finally the weavers started coming back. We taught it in school, we had evening gatherings, and we'd gather materials. I had people coming here to the house to sit down [and learn]. ... With the kids in school, we'd start out maybe with twenty to twenty-three students. When I ended up, I had two left, but the two that stuck with it, they're really good weavers today. Some of them would come back [to it] later.*

An early effort to merge pottery and basketry occurred in May 1955 when the Hoopa Pottery Guild set up a display at the Eureka Hobbies-in-Action show at the Eureka Women's Clubhouse. Lizzie Smith and Josephine Peters, both wearing basket caps, demonstrated basketry behind a table arrayed with Guild member pottery. The press called this "one of the most fascinating exhibits at the show" (Peters 1950s–1970s).

Two years earlier, in 1953, the guild created a float for Hoopa's Fourth of July celebration, atop which Alice Bruce presided in full dance regalia. At the back of the float, they made gigantic representations of a pottery teapot and pottery teacup adorned with basketry designs (Peters 1950s–1970s).

In 1966, the Hoopa Pottery Guild hosted its first Art and Pottery Exhibit in the guild's new studio. Evelyn Osborne, the project chair, who came with her husband to work in the mills, reported "some 150 persons ... in attendance," some traveling to Hoopa from the Coast. In addition to the pottery display, and a display of Nettie McKinnon's basketry collection, Hoopa high school students showed their art, and, as a result, were invited to also show at Eureka's Hobart Gallery. Mrs. Richard (Elsie Gardner) Ricklefs displayed regalia and Mrs. Fern Gibson, a non-Indian, showed fabric painting. Josephine Peters, Vivien Hailstone, and Leona Alameda (Yurok) were among those credited with the exhibit's success.

Holly McClellan (Karuk/Hupa), wearing regalia, was named 1966's Miss Hoopa Pottery Guild. Leona Alameda and Grace Alden (Arcata) presented her with a pottery bust of a Hoopa Indian girl (Peters 1950s–1970s).

Mrs. Ruth Larsen, the guild's 1967 president, announced that the second annual pottery show would occur on May 7. Josephine, guild vice-president at the time, was one of sixteen women who displayed their pottery that day. That same year, pottery classes took place in Hoopa through College of the Redwoods. In 1971, Josephine was elected president. She also served as secretary and treasurer during various years (Peters 1950s–1970s).

Sharing Cultural Traditions at County and State Fairs

Throughout the late 1950s and 1960s, David Risling, Sr. (Chief Su-Worhrom) organized summertime cultural shows for various events, including county and state fairs as far away as Anadarko, Oklahoma. Through these shows, he wanted to dispel the negative images that the print and visual media promulgated about American Indians: *Everybody hated Indians at that time. […] Pop Risling, Vivien's dad, wanted to show people that Indians weren't bad, and that they didn't have to be afraid of them. […] They had a culture. They knew how to do different things.*

Su-Worhrom was a Karuk village where David's grandfather and other family members were the dance givers. The shows David organized focused on northwest California ceremonies, with Vivien narrating, and family members and friends of all ages participating on stage. They also included presentations of Plains cultural traditions and a folk dance. As described by the *Blue Lake Advocate* of August 11, 1966,

> Chief Su-Worhrom has the inheritance rights of his ancestors. He has dedicated his life to the preservation of Indian culture. Chief Su-Worhrom also inherited rights of the Iroquois by a will made to him by Chief Gayandovana, which included his personal ceremonial costume, plus beautifully beaded Eastern costumes, some of the most beautiful in existence. Along with this, Gayandovana willed Su-Worhrom, by Indian law, his songs, dances and representative rights. He was an Iroquois Chief, who spoke and acted for his people from the Atlantic to the Pacific.

David met his Iroquois friend in San Francisco, where he constructed homes for the influx of new residents during World War II. (David Risling, Jr., personal communication with Beverly Oritz, 2003)

Josephine made some of the regalia worn by the performers of the Risling Indian Village Troupe, including the girls' two-parted skirts, war bonnets, Eagle Dance outfits, and the ankle bracelets with bells worn during the hoop dance. She based the out-of-area regalia on dances seen during her travels; she based the war bonnets on photographs in books.

During World War II, the ceremonial dances at Hoopa had been discontinued. As they gradually began anew, Josephine made some of the girls' skirts for them. She also wove basketry caps, which had become scarce.

At the fairs, Josephine set up a sales area for pottery, jewelry, and basketry inside a tipi, the first such public sales effort in her area. She was accompanied by Ella Johnson (Yurok) and/or Nettie McKinnon (Yurok), who demonstrated basketry: *That really drew a good crowd,* Josephine recalls. Her pottery won many prizes in the fairs, including those at Ferndale and Redwood Acres (see Figure 1.18).

Once, in Ferndale, a group of 4-H children threw rocks at the troupe's tents at night. Much to their surprise, they found out that David Rising, Jr., David Risling, Sr.'s son, was the stock show judge, and tried to apologize. As Josephine explains, *All they saw was cowboys and Indians in the movies, I guess, and the Indians were the bad people.*

An early effort to dispel stereotypes took place at Hoopa in the summer of 1957 when thirty-eight teachers from Sacramento schools joined Sacramento State College students as guests of the Hoopa Valley Tribe. Ernie Marshall, Sr. (Hupa), David Risling, Sr.'s son-in-law, welcomed the participants, stating his hope that the "interest of others might be an incentive to the Hoopa people to start now to preserve their songs, legends and dances before they are forgotten." Elise (Gardner) Ricklefs sang

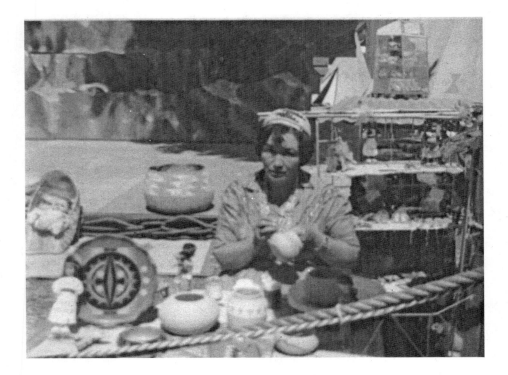

a prayer song. Several men demonstrated "cards," a local gambling game played with sticks (aka Indian cards). Susie Little (Yurok), through an interpreter, shared a story about the history she witnessed. David Risling, Louis Matilton (Hupa), and several dancers shared ceremonial traditions. Lizzie Smith demonstrated basketry. Josephine, identified as the "youngest basket weaver in Hoopa Valley" by Betty Allen, who reported the event, also demonstrated basketry. The Hoopa Pottery Guild had a display, put together by Mrs. Helen Amos, Mrs. Esther Cullaugh (Round Valley/Covelo/Hupa), Mrs. Ernie (Rosalind) Marshall (Karuk/Yurok/Hoopa), Sr., and Mrs. Leslie Rice, who came to Hoopa with her husband to work in the mills.

From June 14 through June 17, 1962, about thirty members of the Risling troupe traveled to the Colusa County Fair to make cultural presentations. Ella Johnson demonstrated basketry, and Josephine displayed her pottery (see Figure 1.19) (Peters 1950s–70s).

The Ferndale Enterprise of August 18, 1966, documented a troupe presentation at the Humboldt County Fair, where Ella and Josephine teamed up again. Josephine's three-year-old daughter Tamara performed on stage with twenty-four other dancers. Five others helped backstage and in the camp.

The Revival of Basketry

On June 19, 1959, Vivien Hailstone opened I-Ye-Quee, a gift shop through which locally created objects were sold. The event was commemorated by a basket, made by Ella Johnson, with the opening date woven in. The store provided an outlet for Josephine's and others' creations, including Josephine's sister-in-law Lee Marshall (Yurok/Karuk) and mother-in-law Daraxa Peters (Yurok/Karuk). In addition to basketry and pottery, the women created stunning jewelry, all inspired by the old-time ways, but, at the same time, reflective of individual creativity and contemporary influences (see Figure 1.20).

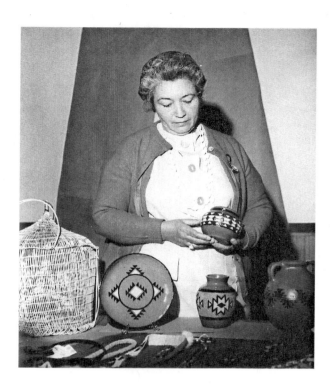

Figure 1.19.
Josephine Peters with some of her pottery. On left, "people sitting around fire" design. Other designs are Josephine's own innovations. Photo courtesy Josephine Peters.

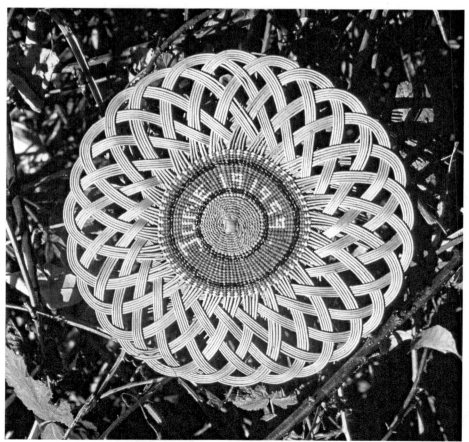

Figure 1.20.
Basket made by Ella Johnson to celebrate the opening of Vivien Hailstone's I-Ye-Quee gift shop in Hoopa Valley. Photo by Beverly Ortiz.

Josephine was the first to use gray pine nuts in her jewelry. Previously, pine nut beads had solely been used as a decorative element of the skirts worn during ceremonial dances.

At first they tried to stop me from making beads, but I didn't listen to them. I just went ahead. Pretty soon everybody was doing it. So many Indians here didn't have enough money, so I started making jewelry and pottery to show them that they could pick this up and do things to earn money.

Lee, Daraxa, and Josephine developed the idea for basketry medallions on bolo ties while working on woven table mats: *"We just made one ... It was fast money stuff."* Maggie Bennett Grant made beads for her daughter; Josephine's nephew loom-beaded chokers.

As the years passed, the creative exchange of ideas among the various artisans, including Vivien, resulted in many new and unique objects, at once beautiful and utilitarian, a statement of the past merging with the present: hide keychains decorated with abalone pendants, trade beads and dentalia; cigarette lighters encased in open-twined basketry; basketry rattles filled with pennies and store-bought olive shells; basketry and beaded barrettes; beaded earrings with abalone pendants; basketry medallions hung with trade beads, pine nuts, abalone, and dentalia, sometimes the smooth, old-time species that had been traded from Vancouver Island, more usually the ribbed species, imported for sale from the Mediterranean. Braided beargrass also became a decorative element (Ortiz 1988: 28).

For basketry and beargrass braiding to continue, hazel and beargrass needed to be burned. Without fire, beargrass blades grow relatively sharp and stiff; hazel bushes lack the straight, flexible shoots that provide the foundation for a shapely basket. In the old days, people set the necessary, low burning fires in the fall; in modern times one risked a jail term to do so. Now weavers work in cooperation with their tribes, private land holders, and the Forest Service to conduct the necessary burns (Ortiz 1988, 1998, 1999, field data).

In 1966, the newly formed Yurok-Karok-Hoopa Weavers of the Klamath-Trinity Arts and Crafts Association announced their plans to begin teaching basketry to all interested individuals at the Hoopa Pottery House on Loop Road north of the Presbyterian Church. Registration occurred at the I-Ye-Quee Gift Shop. Ella Johnson served as instructor and Josephine Peters as associate instructor.

The program will be assisted financially by grants from the Save The [sic] Children Foundation and the Indian Arts and Crafts Board. These grants were made possible through the efforts of Edward Malin, arts and crafts consultant to the Bureau of Indian Affairs. (Sharp 1966)

According to a press release by an unidentified writer printed in a local newspaper (see Figure 1.21),

Historically the art of basketry, as practiced by the members of the Yurok, Karok, and Hoopa tribes of this area, reached its zenith as a skill and craft. This art was purposeful as well as ornamental and was a tremendous influence on the culture of these people. These artful skills and crafts produced ceremonial baskets, water tight [sic] baskets, baskets for food gathering and sifting, and many other uses. Each with its own design, purpose and decorations. Each constructed by a talented and skilled artist with the pride that goes with excellence.

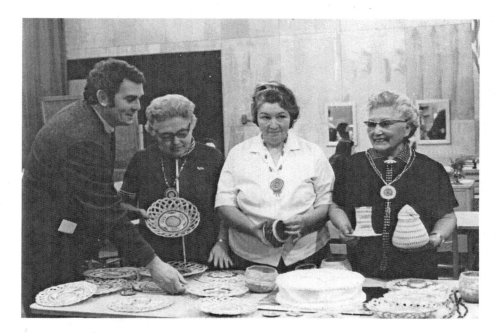

Figure 1.21.
Ken Allen, a local teacher, Vivien Hailstone with student's basket, Josephine VanLandingham (Peters), with basket she made, and Ella Johnson with baskets she made, 1970. Photo courtesy Albert Hailstone and Kathy Wallace from the Vivien Hailstone collection.

Time has wrought severe changes in this priceless art of basketry. Our people had to abandon their way of life, their former skills and become like Europeans. The passage of time continually brings changes in our ways and our thinking. However, we realize that although we must learn the white man's ways we still must be ourselves and preserve our songs, dances, art and skills that are representative of our heritage and culture.

Laws as well as time contributed to the decline of the art of basket weaving. The Forest Service laws prevented the practice of burning specific areas where the particular grasses grew that were necessary for the weaving of the baskets. Without this annual burning and the resulting new growth of these particular grasses and shoots, the raw materials simply were not available for continuing this art. Only recently, my family, local people and our friends throughout the state expended a great deal of time and effort to correct this law that was so damaging to our culture. We are now permitted the privilege of gathering materials from forests and public domain lands.

As a result of these conditions we began to turn to pottery made from clay that is native to this area. We were gradually being forced to this transfer of our skills, talents and art. As our interest in pottery grew a group of ladies formed a pottery guild in 1951. This guild created lots of interest and a pottery house was constructed. The skills steadily improved and soon the projects created by the guild members were winning many awards at local and state fairs. These award winning exhibits contributed in no small way to the recognition of our skills but also as an addition to our economy.

This time nature attempted to hasten the departure of our culture by completely destroying our guild building and many homes as well as countless artifacts and treasured relics of our past during the great flood of 1964. However, the oldest mission church in Hoopa, the Presbyterian Church, realized the importance of the guild building and the purpose of its organization and thus felt that they could help most by building a new pottery house.

We the members of the Pottery Guild have recently revised our by-laws to include any other forms of local arts and crafts. This was the next step to revive the nearly lost art of basket weaving.

We are now organizing a program to teach the art of basketry, which includes the selection of raw materials, treatment of raw materials, the techniques of weaving and design.

We presently plan to begin our lessons about the middle of November 1966 and our new [*sic*] formed group will be called the Yurok-Karok-Hoopa Weavers. (Peters 1950s–1970s)

Class members: Susan Burdick, Mary Koontz, Lucille Bruce, Zona Ferris, Florence Whitehead, Bertha Mitchell, Kim Yerton, Karis Whitman, Lorna Dodge, Ellen Blake, Anita Brown, Ida Jean Campbell, Elaine Gilbert, Mary Ullum, LaVerne Glaze, Helen Jordan, Bernice Beaver, Lucille McLaughlin, Helen Pole, Elizabeth Marshall, Lizette Davis, Karen Hoffman, Dorothy McCollum, Susan Van Kirk, Darlene Gray, Nancy Jordan, Mildred Nixon, Virginia Stuart, Marilyn Colegrove, Charlene Colegrove, and Elaine Saxon (Kellems 1970).

And so it was that the first class commenced on November 9 at 2 p.m., and the second one the same day at 7 p.m. (Peters 1950s–1970s). June Bosworth (1967: 11), a participant in the initial series of classes, whose husband worked for the Bureau of Indian Affairs wrote:

Many tribes were represented among the students; Yurok, Karok, Hupa, Wiyot, Sioux, Pomo, Wintoon, Pueblo, and San Juan.

Some of the obstacles Mrs. Hailstone and her teachers had to overcome were difficult. The reeds and branches used in weaving of the baskets were not easy to come by. Many miles were walked, many streams were waded, the annual "burning" to obtain the new growth of special grasses and shoots had to be done. All of this had to be completed before the reeds and branches could be gathered and prepared into kits for the first lesson. Finally to the surprise and delight of many of the students, Mrs. Hailstone informed us that the reeds and bundles were prepared but she was still looking for one more very necessary item—a porcupine! We were all encouraged to keep an eye out for a porcupine; for his quills were to be dyed and woven into the design of the baskets. ...

The baskets had to be exact, the weaving had to be done just so, or you found yourself starting all over again. The nimble fingers of Mrs. Johnson and Mrs. Peters made it look so easy, but there were many sighs and groans as some of the students were told to "pull it out and start all over."

With a twinkle in her eye Mrs. Johnson would tell us, "Now you want to do it right, don't you?" Soon our groans turned to smiles of delight as our baskets finally began to take shape. ...

We were told that the U.S. Forest Service had assisted this program by the controlled burning of hazel bush; of the blue willow sticks that had been peeled and bleached. The spruce roots had to be cooked, split and stripped. ...

Klamath-Trinity Fine Arts Center is proud to have been able to assist in this program. The Save the Children Federation from New Mexico and the Indian Arts and Crafts Board office in Washington, D.C. through the counseling and advice of Edward Malin had brought to this area a renewed interest in the "art of basket weaving."

On May 30, 1967, Vivien organized a cultural program for the Del Norte Historical Society's monthly meeting, including Frank Douglas (Yurok), Ella John-

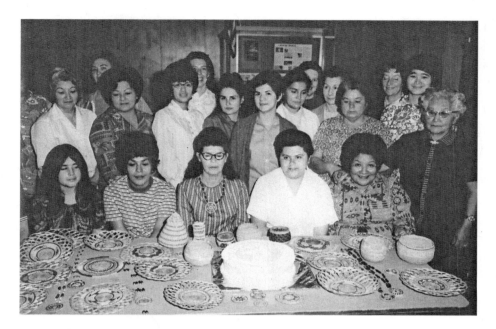

Figure 1.22.
Josephine VanLandingham (Peters) on left and Ella Johnson (on right) with students in basketry class, December 1970. Photo courtesy Josephine Peters.

son, and Amelia Brown (Smith River) presenting songs, Vivien discussing the history of basketry, Ella a demonstration of weaving, and Josephine a presentation about the materials in and functions of the displayed baskets, all woven by Ella (Peters 1950s–1970s). That same year, Josephine entered her work in several exhibitions and shows. As reported by *The Klam-Ity Kourier* on January 17, 1968,

For those who continually bemoan the fact that the native Indian arts are dead, Josephine "Jo" Peters would give a solid argument. Jo is a Karok Indian, daughter of Mr. and Mrs. Frank Grant, Sr., of Somes Bar. She has been a member of the Hoopa Pottery Guild since 1952 and is also a member of the Klamath-Trinity Hoopa Basket Weavers.

In 1967, Jo Peters entered specimens of her work in the National Indian Art Exhibit at Scottsdale, Arizona; the Gallup, New Mexico, Centennial; the Sacramento State Fair; and the First Biennial Exhibit of American Indian Arts at Washington, D.C.

Among her many awards, Mrs. Peters won the Qualla Arts and Crafts Mutual Inc., [sic] award of $50 for Basketry at the Washington, D.C. exhibit and second prize for Pottery exhibited at the 1967 State Fair at Sacramento.

It is hoped that the recognition received by Mrs. Peters will encourage more of the Indian people to produce and exhibit more of their native handcraft which, while not a lost art, certainly has fewer followers today than in the past.

With some difficulty, basketry classes were arranged at Hoopa, beginning in the fall of 1970, through College of the Redwoods extension services. As explained by Vivien Hailstone to Ann Kellems (1970) about the importance and success of the first College of the Redwoods class, which had thirty-one students (see Figure 1.22),

Four people came from Orleans, one from Eurkea [sic], four from Weitchpec and others from all over the Klamath-Trinity area. This class is one that seemed to really meet the needs of the people in this area. ...

We feel that Indian Arts should have a permanent place in the school system.

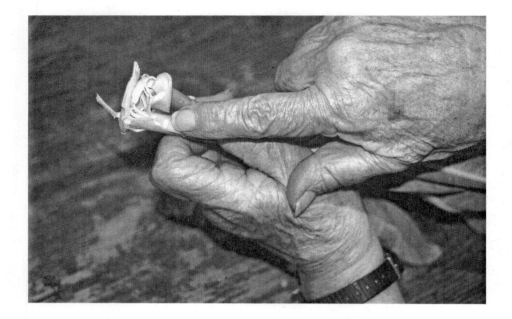

Until instructors of these classes became certified as "eminent persons," they had to accept minimum wage as "assistants" to credentialed art "instructors" who merely took attendance. Josephine Grant Peters received her Community College Provisional Credential to teach "Indian Arts and Crafts" at College of the Redwoods, on July 30, 1972, and again on September 16, 1975. Now extension courses are no longer necessary, as teaching takes place throughout all levels of area schools, and at summertime basket camps (Ortiz 1988: 29; credential documents in possession of Josephine Peters).

In March 2003, LaVerne Glaze (Karuk) described the importance of Josephine's knowledge of basketry to herself and other weavers, and the fond memories that Josephine's plant knowledge engenders.

> I will always be thankful to Josephine for her unselfishness in helping weavers and gatherers with any questions they may have. For me, all it ever took was a brief phone call and Jo would give me a solution to my concern or problem. We did not grow up together, but it seems I've known her most of my life. She has helped me many times with our basket camp, sharing her knowledge of medicinal plants, basket materials and regalia.
>
> We shared stories of gathering milkweed when we were young. We'd put the milk from the plant on the old wood stove in a container and warm it. When cooled, we used it as chewing gum [Figure 1.23]. I don't recall a lot of flavor, but it made for a lot of chewing. (Personal communication, with Beverly Ortiz, March 2003.)

Josephine Establishes Red Wing Indian Handcrafts

Josephine opened a shop, Red Wing Indian Handcrafts, in the late 1960s. She named the shop for a popular song, Red Wing, which her father used to play on his violin: *I always liked that song.*[8]

The song was written by Thurland Cattaway, an Englishman, who came to north Iowa in 1906, where he heard folklore about an "Indian Princess" named Red Wing, whose father was reputedly a chief.[9] Chattaway met composer Kerry Mills in New York City's Tin Pan Alley, and they collaborated on the song, which was recorded for the first time for the Edison Wax Cylinder Company in 1907. Eventually, the lyrics "wandered from the melody," and Red Wing became a popular fiddle tune.[10] The melody later became the inspiration for Woody Guthrie's "Union Maid."[11]

The genesis of Red Wing Indian Handcrafts resides with the pottery Josephine sold at state fairs. The business became formalized in the late 1960s when Harvey Orcutt (Yurok), a professional truck driver, moved a trailer near Josephine's home and created the Rock Shop Museum. There he displayed rocks and petrified wood, the tangible result of his lapidary hobby. Harvey also set up a workshop inside, where he polished stones, then created rings, bolo ties, and other wearable art for sale.

Josephine displayed a wide variety of cultural objects at the Rock Shop Museum, including basketry, basketry materials, dentalia, a dugout, and wood carvings. Josephine, Grace Davis (Karuk), Madeline Davis (Karuk), Daisy Dick, Lena Fisher (Yurok), Jessie Hancorn (Blue Lake), Florence Harrie (Karuk), Patricia Hunsucker (Yurok), Stella Jake (Yurok), Josephine James (Yurok), Ella Johnson (Yurok), Eleonore Logan (Yurok), Bonita Masten (Yurok), Sadie McAuley (Karuk), Sadie McCovey (Yurok), Nettie McKinnon (Yurok), Nettie Moore (Yurok), Amy Peters (Yurok), Minnie Reeves (Hupa/Redwood Creek), Sarah Smoker (Yurok), and Daisy Soctish (Hupa) wove the baskets. Daisy Dick and Jessie Hancorn, both of Blue Lake, were among the few who still had the 111 chin tattoos.

Josephine rounded out her cultural collection with fans and others objects sent from the South Pacific by her brother Wayne, Chief Petty Officer in the U.S. Navy. A trailer addition, which expanded the museum, became the home of Red Wing Indian Handcrafts, where Josephine sold pottery, baskets, and jewelry made by her and others (*Klam-Ity Kourier* 1969; Josephine Peters, personal communication, June 6, 2005).

School groups and other interested people toured the museum. When the tribe established its own museum in the Hoopa Valley shopping center, Josephine closed her museum and began operating Red Wing out of her home. She donated the museum's contents to the Hoopa Museum, China Flat Museum (Willow Creek), Eureka Historical Museum, and the Jesse Peter Memorial Museum (Santa Rosa).

An Unwavering Commitment to Education

Education was a Grant and Brazille family tradition, with Josephine following in the footsteps of Ellen Brazille Grant and Susan Brazille, who chose to share their cultural knowledge with linguists Roland B. Dixon and J. P. Harrington, anthropologist C. Hart Merriam, and ethnomusicologist Helen Roberts. For Josephine, the imperative to share and to educate whenever and wherever called on to do so has been an innate outflow of her giving and patient nature and her keen desire to ensure that the cultural skills the elders so generously shared with her would not only survive into the future, but flourish. In 2004, Deborah McConnell described Josephine's success in achieving this goal.

I have known Josephine Peters since I was a child and our friendship has grown throughout the years. She has a wealth of knowledge about medicinal plants, dressmaking, and basketry and I have often found myself seeking her advice.

Josephine has helped to preserve Northwestern cultural arts such as ceremonial dressmaking and basketry. In the late 1980s, I attended a ceremonial dressmaking class taught by her. Her warm and thoughtful nature helped me, a painfully bashful, young mother, feel at ease about making a ceremonial dress for my daughter. The class met once a week for several months and during that time I grew more and more attached to her because of her unique way of teaching. Once when I was braiding beargrass for my daughter's ceremonial dress, Josephine asked me to show her how to braid grass because it had been a while since she braided grass and forgot how to. As I look back, I think that she was trying to spark my interest in teaching because since then I have also helped young ladies make ceremonial dresses.

Josephine has a gift of making people feel good about their responsibilities and I appreciate and respect her honest, unassuming good nature and am sure that other people who know her feel the same. (Personal communication with Beverly Ortiz, April 21, 2004) [See Figure 1.24]

Over many decades, Josephine has taught, lectured, and demonstrated in countless locales, and participated in numerous museum exhibitions. She has traveled widely to sell her jewelry and that of others at fairs, parks, and conferences. Classes have included those at College of the Redwoods, Hayward State University (now CSU East Bay), Humboldt State University, and UC Riverside, as well as locally, through Indian Education and Johnson O'Malley programs. Lectures and demonstrations have included the Humboldt County Historical Society, the Fortuna Folklife Festival, the California Indian Basketweavers Association, the Heard Museum, and the National Folklife Festival in Washington, DC. Exhibitions have included a showing of Josephine's baskets, regalia, jewelry, and pottery at the San Diego Museum of Man in 1995. Annually, in the late fall and early winter, Josephine sold cultural objects at the State Indian Museum, Hoopa Christmas Bazaar, and in Redding.

True to her commitment to education, Josephine attended the first ever meeting of the Hoopa Valley Indian Education Program of the Klamath-Trinity Unified School District, established under the auspices of the Title IV Act. Fifty other people also attended the meeting, which was held on November 25, 1974. Josephine was elected to serve on the program's ten-member Parents Committee. She later joined the Continuation Grant Committee, which was responsible for acting "on suggestions made … in developing needs, goals, objectives and a budget for the 1975–76 project." She remained active in the program throughout the 1970s, attending meetings regularly, serving on other Continuation Grant Committees, and serving as one of several resource people who conducted cultural activities as part of the program, such as a Third Grade Exchange Day with McKinleyville students.

By 1976, Hoopa Valley Indian Education Program students were receiving instruction from Josephine and other local cultural practitioners in a diversity of cultural skills and the arts in general, including Native American design, local basketry traditions, language, and ceremonial tradition, and sacred narratives and other stories, "so that they may be able to appreciate the fine oral tradition and history of the Native American people." They were also taught ancestral games that emphasize "the social structure of tribes and intertribal associations," taught about ancestral interactions with the local landscape by "local people who still recognize the value of being in harmony with nature," and exposed to other cultural traditions designed to "develop an awareness of our heritage and its valuable contributions to our society."[12]

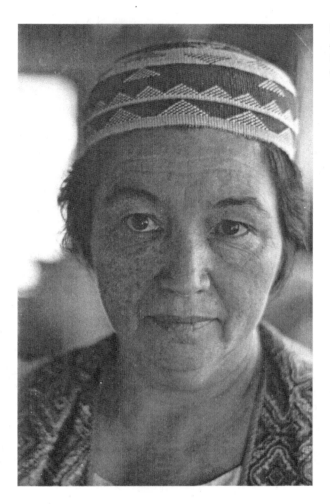

Figure 1.24.
Josephine wearing basketry hat
made by Ella Johnson. Photo
courtesy Josephine Peters.

The goals of these varied cultural initiatives, as stated in a 1976 Indian Education Program continuation grant application in Josephine's possession, mirror the goals that underpinned decades of cultural activities and educational programs in the Hoopa Valley—pride and understanding. As such, several are well worth quoting:

Respect for Indian cultural traditions. . . .

Understanding of special problems that Indian students face in a multi-ethnic society. . . .

Raise the educational, vocational, and economic aspirations of Indian students. . . .

Improvement among teachers and other school staff in the quality of their relationships with students and their overall understanding of the local Indian culture. . . .

Promotion of higher expectations for educational achievement within the school staff, students and community. . . .

An increased knowledge of available resources and instructional strategies appropriate to Native American students.

As another forum for education, this time about community issues, in December 1978 *Common Sense*, a biweekly newspaper, was launched in the Hoopa Valley: "*Common Sense* originated from the need to inform people about decisions that were being made that directly affected them. The first issues were paid for from private donations of a few individuals that believed in the 'right of the people to know'" (Kelsey 1981: 6).

Josephine volunteered to assist with layout of the nascent newspaper, and in January 1981 she became a board member.[13] Her contributions reached their zenith in the August 3, 1981, issue, a thirty-two-page pictorial that featured late 1800s through early 1900s Klamath–Trinity River area history. Subscriptions had grown to 252 and over-the-counter sales to 1,050.[14] Photographs contributed by Josephine ranged from 1920s stick game players in Orleans to portraits of Native peoples of the Trinity River area, including Weitchpec and Somes Bar, all from her personal collection. On September 12, 1980, *Common Sense* became a nonprofit under the aegis of The Hoopa Newspaper Project, with Josephine serving as project secretary.

Josephine has been called on to assist with and participate in countless tribal events, where her impact has been deep and lasting. As recalled in 2005 by Stacey McConnell (Yurok),

> We had what we call a GONA or Gathering of Native Americans at Hoopa. This was a healing ceremony for our community, to be taught to our people by other Native Americans, and all the elders were invited. I was a helper, and I got to help Jo. With her status, being able to help her was more than enough for me, but on the last day, we all had to make beads for a give away.
>
> This occurred in a room with 75 people, and for most of the day, everybody made necklaces, earrings, key chains, etc. Jo watched me make earrings that day. I was nervous, thinking that because of her talent, in her eyes those earrings must look amateurish and sloppy. That night, before dinner, there was a table set up, and all the jewelry was placed there. Our give away had begun.
>
> All the elders were to go first, with Jo first of all. She got her cane and walked all around those tables, looking and searching. All of the sudden her eyes got big and sparkly. She found what she was looking for. Out of all that jewelry, she chose my little pair of earrings. She held them up, searched the circle and found my face. She nodded her head and winked. This made my whole day, week and month. I felt a peace established in my heart due to this special woman with her ancient ways, like my ancestors. (Personal communication, with Beverly Ortiz, July 16, 2005).

Josephine has also served as a cultural consultant to museums, institutions, and agencies, including the Forest Service. Ken Wilson vividly remembers his first meeting with her, when she served as a cultural consultant on traditional gatherers' herbicide concerns:

> I first met Josephine in the mid-1980s while conducting interviews with basketweavers regarding proposed herbicide spraying in timber plantations. The interviews were set up by Joy Sundberg (Yurok), with Yurok, Tolowa, and Karuk weavers. The Forest Service was aware of weavers' concerns about placing basketry materials in their mouths that might be contaminated with herbicides. The intent of the interviews was to identify timber plantations proposed for spraying and ascertain if they were in areas of traditional gathering.

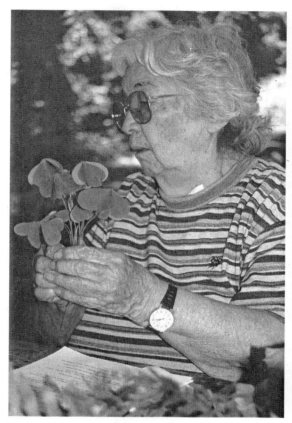

Figure 1.25.
Josephine sharing redwood sorrel at Following the Smoke. Photo by Beverly Ortiz.

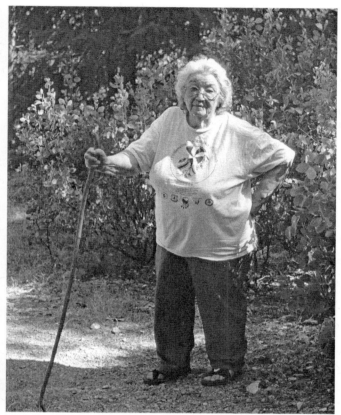

Figure 1.26.
Josephine standing amidst manzanita across the river from the Old Home Place, August 30, 2001. Photo by Beverly Ortiz.

As soon as I met Josephine, I knew I was in the presence of a person with a unique knowledge of plants and how to utilize these plants to heal and help people. To this day, I remember watching her open her suitcase and take out each plant or medicine, explaining how it was utilized. I thought of her as a country doctor with her suitcase being her doctor's "black bag." I was in awe of this remarkable woman when I first met her. I continue to be in awe of Josephine. (Personal communication with Beverly Ortiz, July 13, 2005) [see Figure 1.25]

Josephine has been interviewed for several tribal projects, and featured in numerous articles and books. Her knowledge is also preserved in the archives of the late Wayne State University anthropologist Arnold Pilling, with whom she had a decades-long friendship. Many museums have collected her work, including the Smithsonian, Heard, Hearst, and Qualla Arts.

Following is a chronological sampling of some of the publications for which Josephine has served as a consultant, or in which she is featured: LaPena 1987, Reese Bullen Gallery 1991, Cohodas 1997, Johnson and Marks 1997, Ortiz 1999, Roberts 1999, Marshall 1999, Navarro 2000/01, Buckley 2002,[15] and now this book (see Figure 1.26).

NOTES

1. Unless otherwise indicated, all information in this chapter comes from taped and written interviews and conversations conducted with Josephine Peters by Beverly Ortiz from 2001 through 2005.

2. For Karuk sacred narratives, see Angulo and Freeland (1931), Bright (1954, 1957), Graves (1929), Harrington (1931, 1932a), and Kroeber and Gifford (1980).

3. These are tubular mollusk shells, originally traded from Vancouver Island, and now largely obtained from Asia.

4. Ellen Brazille and her sister Susan served as cultural consultants for Roland B. Dixon in 1903, Jaime de Angulo, who recorded Konimihu words, in 1928, and Helen H. Roberts (date unknown), who recorded songs. They also worked with J. P. Harrington in 1928. Harrington returned to his work with Susan in 1933, during which time her brother Henry and son Johnny were present (Heizer 1967: 241–242; Mills 1985: II/29–48; Silver 1978: 224).

5. As elaborated in this section of the manuscript, Josephine's plant uses are multifaceted. For more about Karuk plant use, see Baker (1981), Davis and Hendryx (1991) Harrington (1932b) Lake (2007), and Schenck and Gifford (1952).

6. This information about talking to plants and songs was shared by Josephine during a January 27, 1976, lecture at California State University East Bay, for an anthropology course taught by Lowell John Bean. Course notes courtesy student Mary Lou Wilcox.

7. Josephine had another stroke at age 37 or 38 and another mild one when she was 80.

8. To view the lyrics, see www.fortunecity.com/tinpan/parton/2/redwing.html. To purchase a recent recording of the song, contact the Pioneer Music Museum, www.oldtimemusic.tipzu.com/pioneer-music-museum.

9. The song tells the story of a young Indian woman who falls in love with an Indian man who is killed in battle. The motif of an American Indian love story involving the children of chiefs that ends in tragedy is widespread among non-Indians. It arises, for instance, in non-Indian folklore about Mount Diablo, California (Ortiz 1989).

10. Bob Everhart, president of the National Traditional Country Music Association and curator for the Pioneer Music Museum in Iowa, personal communication, June 20, 2005.

11. See www.unionsong.com/u023.html.

12. Title IV Meeting Minutes and Continuation Grant applications in possession of Josephine Peters.

13. Kelsey 1981: 6; January 21, 1981, Hoopa Newspaper Project Board of Directors Minutes, copy in possession of Beverly Ortiz.

14. May 22, 1991 report to the Board of Directors, copy in possession of Josephine Peters.

15. Buckley's characterization of Josephine's doctoring on page 107 is incorrect. She did not seek doctoring powers in the high country.

CHAPTER TWO

Gathering Ethics

Once you have identified a plant that you would like to gather for medicinal use, it is important to make sure that you will not negatively affect wild plant populations by overharvesting. According to Bryan Colegrove, who helps Josephine gather plants for medicines,

> Josephine instructed us to take a little bit from here, a little bit from there. Just take what you need, not any more... Before you go out [to gather], you have to show respect. You have to go with an open mind and a clean heart, just like with basketweaving... If you don't have an open mind and a clean heart, then the stuff that you gather may not be as strong, may not even work at all.

Here are some general guidelines to consider when gathering plants from the wild.

Only Gather What You Will Use

Take good care of what you do gather. Share with people who need it and can't get out to gather the plants themselves. If you are able, gather from areas that are more difficult to access so elders can gather from places that are easier to get to. When gathering leaves or flowers, cut branches from several individual plants rather than pulling the plant up by the roots, which will kill the plant. When gathering from shrubs, take less than five percent of an individual plant.

Gather Plants from Large Populations

Take small amounts from several stands to minimize your impact on the plant population. For long-lived plants, a good general rule is to take less than one twentieth, or five percent, of the plant material from a given site. It's typical for just one percent of a plant's seeds to survive in nature, so, if you are gathering annuals, spread the seeds at the site if possible. Get to know the plants and adjust your gathering methods to make sure that the plants thrive.

Only Gather Common Plants

Some common plants have rare relatives that that resemble them closely. Be certain of plant identification before you harvest.

Figure 2.1.
Josephine watering herbs and
flowers in her home garden.
Photo by Beverly Ortiz.

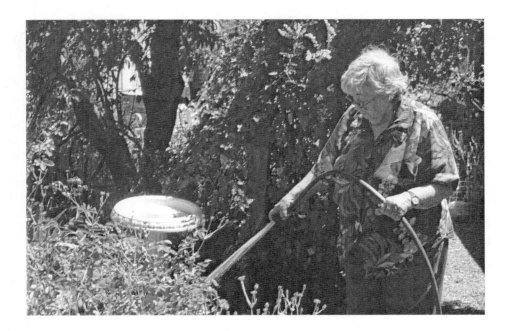

Avoid Gathering Frequently from the Same Place

Also encourage other people not to gather from the same place. Slow-growing plants can easily be overharvested, especially if the root is the part used.

Bring Wild Plants into Your Garden

Gather seeds or cuttings to grow in your garden so that you don't have to keep finding new places to gather from in the wild.

Learn About Invasive Exotic Species

Give back to the earth by removing invasive species from your gathering sites. Be aware that you are spreading seeds as you move from one place to another; if you have seeds of invasive weeds in your shoes, try to remove them as best you can before going to another gathering site.

Gather Only from Healthy Plants

Do not gather from areas infected with Sudden Oak Death or Port Orford cedar root disease. Learn to recognize the symptoms of these diseases and take care not to spread them. Port Orford cedar root disease can be spread on shoes and car tires. Sudden Oak Death can infect many species of native plants, and can be spread by moving infected plants, including firewood. For the most up-to-date information on the innumerable species affected by Sudden Oak Death and how you can prevent its spread, see www.suddenoakdeath.org, the website of the California Oak Mortality Task Force. At the site, you can sign up to receive a monthly report on developments pertaining to this disease, including monitoring, management, and other related activities. The site also contains information on tribal issues related to the disease, including guidelines for plant gatherers.

Learn the Rules Governing Plant Gathering

Obtain permission from private landowners, and learn the regulations governing public lands where you gather. For more information, see the California Indian Basketweavers Association website at www.ciba.org.

It is important to consider the overall impact of various people who gather in the same areas. Be sensitive to the fact that you may have found a site considered to be someone else's territory. If the site looks tended or recently harvested, keep looking for another spot to gather. On national forest lands, permits are given for some commercial collection of medicinal plants, of greenery for the floral industry, and mushrooms. Find out who else is gathering in your area, where they tend to gather, and learn to recognize the impact of these different types of wild plant use.

For more information about gathering ethics and how to propagate native plants, see Emery (1988), Rose, et al. (1998), and Tilford (1998).

CHAPTER THREE

Herbal Medicines and Native Plant Foods

INTRODUCTION

On the following pages, you'll find general information about how Josephine Peters gathers and processes plants, along with recipes for making them into teas (decoctions), blood purifiers, cleansers, gargles, inhalants, rinses for hair, soaks, washes, capsules, poultices, pastes, plasters, salves, syrups, cough drops, and various foods. Next, you'll find a complete list of the medicinal plants Josephine uses, with in-depth information about how she uses each one.

Josephine's own words have been incorporated into the text in italic typeface. Her voice should remind you that this is a very personal ethnobotany, one which represents a lifetime of learning and thinking about plants, and taking and prescribing plant remedies, by a particular woman with a particular history. Josephine's words may help you access, as well, the utter joy of traveling with her through the landscape she knows so intimately, learning about the plants firsthand. Finally, a small measure of her inestimable good humor, practicality, forthrightness, and generosity will hopefully shine through.

PLANT GATHERING

Josephine gathers most of her medicinal herbs after the first full moon in April: *We don't have much wintertime sun, and we've got to have the sun on the plant for a certain length of time to get the strength in it. It's the only time we ever went to gather, except the roots. Then we wait until the plant goes back to seed.*

Until the plants have died back, the roots lack strength. Before this, as Josephine puts it, *There's nothing in it.*

Josephine continues to gather all but her roots until the plants start dying back—about August in her area. She cautions that flowers take some of the plant's strength, although this isn't a consideration in cases where the medicinal qualities reside in the flower itself, as with chamomile, grindelia and St. John's wort.

When gathering, Josephine approaches the plants she harvests in a respectful, thoughtful way, preparing her mind for the plant's ability to heal. As she explains: *When you go out and gather an herb, you've got to pray to it, that it's going to help.*

Josephine's gathering tools include gardening scissors and pruning shears, a shovel, and an assortment of paper bags and string, to bundle those herbs with relatively rigid stalks, like grindelia. In the old days, local Native peoples gathered and sorted herbs in baskets. Today, paper bags offer an apt substitute, but one should never use plastic, which can contaminate the herbs with chemicals, and cause them to sweat and rot.

When gathering plants, Josephine focuses on locations away from main roads, where cars won't leave dust and chemicals on them.[1] Roots, of course, will pick up some dirt. Once home, Josephine scrubs these with a heavy-bristled brush, the type that has a flat, rectangular wooden handle. To avoid clogging the sink, she does the scrubbing outside, under a hose, with the roots secure in a pan.

Sticky plants, which pick up dust, also need rinsing. Josephine holds the new growth of mountain balm, with the leaves attached to the stem, beneath lukewarm water in her sink, or bundles two or three such tips together, hangs them upside-down from an old peach tree in her front yard, and sprays them with hose water. Outside rinsing is preferable, since the oils can block the sink drain. Josephine dips grindelia tops up and down in a clean metal bucket of water three times until the sticky residue is gone, then hangs them upside-down to dry from her roofed porch, where they're further protected from dust. She ties the bundles according to the amount of herb she plans to use.

DRYING AND STORING

Most medicinal herbs can be used fresh, or dried for winter use. Those with juicy stems, like chickweed, should only be used fresh. Others dry so readily when picked—unless they're growing close to home—that they're never used fresh. When making salves, it's best to use fresh herbs, although, as described below, some of the component herbs can be used dry.

To dry whole plants for tea, tie them into bundles at the base of the stems, then hang them upside down so that, as Josephine says, *the juices won't run out.* When only the flower parts will be used, as with mullein and St. John's wort, lay the flower itself out to dry in a clean place. Lay roots out to dry as well. If they're large, split them in half and with the centers facing up.

Josephine stores dried herbs whole, crushed, or she uses an electric chopper. As a general rule, those herbs that will be used within a year, such as yerba buena, get put in boxes or, more commonly, paper bags, but never plastic, lest they become contaminated with the chemicals. Closeable waxed boxes, akin to those used for restaurant leftovers, work well for the purpose. Herbs that will be stored for more than a year, or that lose their potency relatively quickly, get put in jars. Examples of the latter include angelica tops, Indian tobacco, lobelia, mints, rose hips, and skullcap, as well as dried currants and acorn flour. Josephine stores grapevine (wild grape) sap in jars, but only saves milkweed sap for a few days.

NON-NATIVE PLANTS

This ethnobotany includes several non-native species. Their presence has sometimes resulted from the purposeful introduction of these species into the local area, such as by Chinese miners or by individuals growing them in home gardens. Other species

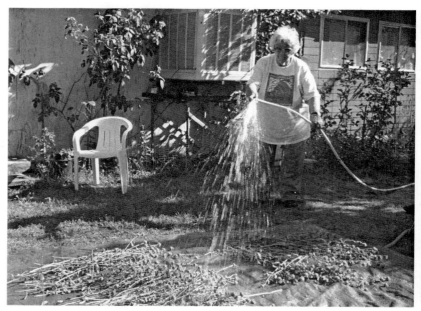

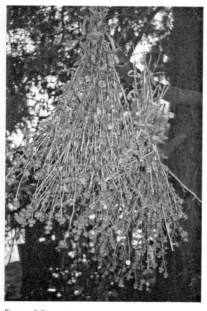

Figure 3.1.
Josephine Peters washing grindelia prior to bundling it at the cut ends, and hanging it up to dry in her Hoopa Valley porch. Photo by Beverly Ortiz, July 20, 2001.

Figure 3.2.
Bundle of grindelia hanging to dry in Josephine's porch. Photo by Beverly Ortiz.

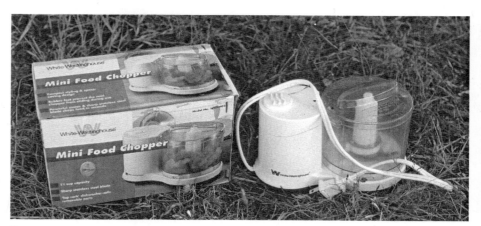

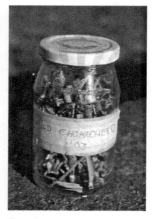

Figure 3.3.
Mini food chopper that Josephine uses today to process her herbs. Photo by Beverly Ortiz.

Figure 3.4.
Dried choke-cherry bark stored in glass jar to preserve its freshness ("strength"). When stored in paper bags, herbs lose their strength within six months. Photo by Beverly Ortiz.

were brought into the area inadvertently, such as in hay bales. Once naturalized, their use spread throughout the local communities, often before Josephine was born.

While the uses of most naturalized plants are relatively new to the Karuk, in some instances the native and domestic species of the same genus work equally well to cure an illness. Examples include garden and native violets (Johnny-jump-ups), wild and domestic geraniums, and native and commercial species of mushrooms. Not all plants with the same common name are related, however. Wild and domestic ginger, for example, aren't even in the same family, but, probably due to a similar medicinal component, have the same smell.

Josephine prescribes several herbs that are neither native nor locally naturalized. These she learned about from the sons of a Chinese herbalist, Indian doctors from Canada, Mexico, the Eastern United States and beyond, and knowledgeable Cahuilla and Pueblo elders. Josephine has some of these herbs, such as gotu kola, shipped in. She obtains others in health food stores. Still others she acquires through in-person visits and exchanges by mail with Indian doctors she has known for years.

TESTING OF MEDICINALS

Some of the medicinal herbs Josephine uses were tested years ago at a laboratory in San Francisco by a gentleman who sought her out. More recently, Hoopa Valley Indian Health Service Clinic staff members arranged for the testing of others. Among the latest findings, dogwood and wild choke-cherry, used by Josephine for heart medicine, lowers high blood pressure. Information acquired from the tests has been incorporated into the descriptions found below.

PREPARATION OF MEDICINALS

The preparation of medicinal teas, salves and syrups involves far more than merely chopping, measuring, mixing, steeping, or simmering. To Josephine, the preparer's, and the patient's, attitude is central: *When you're fixing it and giving it, you've got to pray to it that it's going to help this person. The person's got to be a believer in it, too.*

After the preparation of herbal medicines, the decocted or strained herbs must be disposed of. Most of the time, Josephine throws these among the plants in her yard. Oily or greasy herbs, such as tarweed and mountain balm, can kill garden plants, however, so Josephine adds these to the other weeds, branches and tree limbs in her burn pile. Burning eliminates tarweed seeds, ensuring that the plants don't spread throughout the yard.

TYPES OF MEDICINALS

Teas

When taking a medicinal tea for the first time, you should test for allergic reactions by first drinking only a small amount: about one teaspoon for babies, two teaspoons for children, and a shot glass worth to a quarter cup for adults. Allergic reactions occur within four to six hours; symptoms include vomiting or the development of rashes.

With St. John's wort, Josephine recommends that adults start with half a cup to see how their system will react: *If it rejects it, then you give them something else. A lot of people can't take the same herb... If it doesn't bother them, they can take a cupful.*

It's ordinarily best to prepare each dose of medicinal tea right before taking it. In general, medicinal teas should be relatively light in color, comparable to the strength of the non-medicinal teas one might savor with a meal. When I asked Josephine how she determines the correct dosage, she responded: *It all depends on what I'm giving it for, [and] on the patient and what they can handle.*

Most teas require a teaspoonful of herbs per cup of hot water, or two tablespoons for a quart. For fresh herbs, these amounts are only guidelines, since Josephine adds them based on experience rather than measurement. When using dried herbs, which are less potent than fresh ones, Josephine adds a heaping, rather than level, teaspoon or tablespoonful.

Josephine boils her tea water to sterilize it. She never boils herbs directly in the water, however, even when brewing large amounts, lest they lose too much of their potency. Rather, she advises boiling the water separately, then letting it sit for three or four minutes before pouring it into a container of pre-measured herbs. Josephine recommends the use of bottled water, rather than from the tap, due to the chlorine in most municipal water supplies. As a *"chemical,"* chlorine will contaminate the medicine.

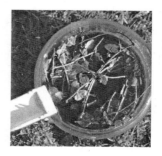

Figure 3.5.
Yerba buena tea steeped in pyrex pot. Photo by Beverly Ortiz.

In a few cases, the boiling water may be poured directly on the herbs. The oily, tar-like residue on the leaves of mountain balm, and the gummy residue on grindelia, are dissolved by boiling water. New fir tips, gathered in the spring and used for treating colds, are somewhat pitchy. Josephine lets these three teas steep for about fifteen to twenty minutes, then strains off the sticky substances through old flour sacks she acquires from bakeries.

To prevent any metal residues from contaminating the water, Josephine boils her tea water in Pyrex or *"granite"* (white-spotted enamel) kettles, never metal. She steeps her herbs in non-metal containers as well, lest some react with the metal. For small dosages, she uses a tea or coffee cup. For large amounts, she uses a glass container, such as quart canning jars or gallon storage jars. Mayonnaise jars, which people save for Josephine, provide a particularly suitable size for brewing batches of herbs. Although Josephine has used crockery, she cautions: *[S]ometimes you don't know what's in the glaze they put on it.*

While the herbs steep, always cover them. Cover teacups with a saucer or lid, or jars with their own lid. Try not to let the herb touch the lid. Let the tea steep for about 20 minutes before taking.

After the tea water has steeped, Josephine strains the herbs out through the flour sack. A few herbs, notably yerba buena and Josephine's dogwood and chokecherry heart medicine, become stronger as they soak, and work more effectively when not strained.

Ideally, medicinal teas should be made fresh each time they're taken. With dosages ranging from half to one cup twice or more a day, however, making teas fresh can be time-consuming. For her own use, Josephine generally makes a pint to a quart at a time, the equivalent of one to two days' worth. She only exceeds a quart when using an herb she uses a lot, like yerba buena. Then she'll steep a gallon.

Many herbs with medicinal qualities have pleasant flavors, and may be savored solely for their agreeable taste. Josephine particularly enjoys pennyroyal, yerba buena, peppermint, spearmint, and Labrador tea. In the case of the latter, she cautions that it isn't good to take too much. She also cautions that pregnant women shouldn't drink pennyroyal, as it can cause an abortion.

Josephine's Pyrex pot holds about ten cups of tea: *When I'm using yerba buena, I make that whole potful, because the kids will drink it up in a day.*

The making of larger batches of medicinal teas depends, for the most part, on how long the tea can be safely and effectively stored in the refrigerator. Mint teas, such as yerba buena and pennyroyal, and blood purifiers, can be stored for Josephine's maximum two weeks.

Some herbal teas—in particular, peach, Labrador tea, mistletoe and skullcap—become toxic if left sitting. Lady slipper root, while not as dangerous as the others, also requires judicious use. In fact, some herbal remedies can be so dangerous to take that the details of their preparation and dosage have been withheld from this book.

Batch sizes also depend on the severity of the illness, how long the tea must be taken, and where the person who will be taking it lives. Josephine makes gallon-sized batches when the tea will keep two weeks and the case is severe. This ensures that her patients will continue taking it. She also makes gallon-sized batches when the tea will keep and her patients live far away, and thus can't easily return for more. She'll give them a quart when they live close by. If they don't, but the tea must be made in small batches, she provides them with a quart's worth, enough herbs to make the needed dosages, and directions for preparing them.

When stored in the refrigerator, the prescribed dosage may be taken hot or cold. Josephine drinks her teas cold in the summertime. In the wintertime, when she wants to take the chill off, she reheats a dosage-worth of tea in the microwave for two minutes. Before the existence of microwaves, she left the tea on the back of her wood-burning heater stove, or heated it on her stove top. When reheating, the tea should be warmed, never boiled.

Josephine generally adds a little heal-all (self heal) to her teas due to the plant's qualities as a blood purifier. She adds about two tablespoons of fresh heal-all per quart of tea. She also adds it to her salves. For ready availability, Josephine planted heal-all in her yard. She recommends placing a little "*root*" in the ground in early spring, at the time of the first rains. The plant will spread from its rhizomes (underground stems).

Some herbal teas may be taken to prevent a cold when you feel one coming on. In such cases, Josephine advises that the tea be taken when it's still "*pretty warm*," as hot as can be tolerated. Take three cups in quick succession throughout the day. The more you take, the more chance you have of preventing a cold.

For the most part, Josephine prescribes medical teas to adults. Babies don't get tea very often, unless they have colic, whooping cough, or a really bad chest cold. Small babies get about three drops from a dropper; alternatively, about five drops in a teaspoon of water. Babies of about a year-and-a-half to a year old can take about one teaspoon. Children through age five get about half a cup. Children of five or six years old get about half a cup of tea diluted to just about half strength, up to three quarters of the standard dose. By the time they're ten, they can take a full cup, like adults.

Blood Purifiers

Josephine uses blood purifiers to cleanse the liver (remove "*poisons*" from the system). Josephine gathers more blood purifiers than other herbs: *We have to purify our blood to get it to help prevent diseases... For some sicknesses we need a lot of that.*

Of the locally available blood purifiers, Josephine prefers Oregon grape and heal-all: *I generally recommend Oregon grape. It's a good one, and it's easier on them.* Although not locally available, Mormon tea is another "*good one,*" that, when available, Josephine rates behind Oregon grape, ahead of heal-all. After these three, Josephine prefers echinacea. Echinacea, which comes in powdered form, wasn't grown in the local area until relatively recently. Goldenseal comes next: *Goldenseal is a good one, but a lot of them can't take it. It's a strong herb.* [....] *With the burdock and the curly dock, it's too nasty to take* [laughs]. When Josephine was able to obtain devil's club along the north coast, she sometimes used it as a blood purifier.

Oregon grape and heal-all may be taken straight through. Goldenseal and burdock can damage the kidneys, so these should only be taken for three or four days, then discontinued for two before resuming. An Indian doctor from back east sends Josephine goldenseal in both the root and powdered forms.

Josephine recommends that blood purifiers be taken annually in the spring. At two cups a day, one in the morning, one in the evening (or half a cup four times a day, as Josephine prefers) adult patients will consume eighty-four cups, or more than five gallons of blood purifiers in a season. For personal use, Josephine brews up a quart at a time. Because blood purifiers aren't harmful in quantity, and to ensure that her patients continue to drink them, Josephine brews larger batches for them, although no more than two weeks' worth should be stored at a time.

As with other herbal medicines, some people may have an allergic reaction to particular blood purifiers. To test for possible allergy, start by taking only half a cup.

Josephine drinks blood purifiers for six weeks in both spring and fall. For those who believe in herbal medicines, she recommends they do the same. Taken in the fall, blood purifiers prevent colds and flu.

Josephine usually steeps a quart (two days' worth) of blood purifier at a time for her own use, storing it in the refrigerator. Oregon grape benefits from being left unstrained in the water during storage, which increases the strength of the tea. Nor does Josephine strain Mormon tea or angelica root (*It* [Mormon tea] *gets pretty strong toward the end).* Echinacea, which comes in powdered form, and goldenseal, which comes in powdered and liquid forms, need not be strained. Pink clover should be. Josephine rarely uses pink clover, which was once common but is now relatively rare. In the wintertime, Josephine warms up her stored blood purifiers; in the summertime she drinks them cold.

In Josephine's experience, the older generation, raised on blood purifiers, take them faithfully in spring and fall. The younger generation tends to wait until they're ailing: *It's the same with eating peppernuts in the fall to keep from getting colds and flu. Some will do it. Some won't.*

Blood purifiers are generally taken by adults, but children with ongoing medical problems, especially drug babies, may benefit from starting earlier. For drug babies born with jaundice, Josephine recommends one teaspoon of blood purifier twice a day in a bottle of milk. She prescribes half a cup three times a day for children with pancreatitis. Twelve is the earliest age that she starts children on a regular course. Teenagers over fifteen years of age may take an adult dose.

Cleansers

Cleansers, most commonly chickweed and miner's lettuce, flush out the system, similar to a physic or some other laxative. These common cleansers grow in the spring, and must be taken fresh. Josephine recommends taking cleansers for two days prior to starting on a blood purifier.

Chew cleansers raw, or add them to a salad or sandwich. It's important to achieve a balance between eating too little or too much: *The old people knew how much to get.* Josephine eats "*a good handful*" twice a day.

In the fall, Josephine relies on fruit to cleanse her system. She has several types of fruit trees in her yard to pick from, but recommends three or four plums or one cup of applesauce as best. Peaches also work well, but *"you've got to eat several."* Avoid fried food.

Gargles

For sore or strep throat, gargle with as strong a tea as can be tolerated. Josephine recommends making a quart at a time. Put a handful of plant material in a quart jar. Boil water in a separate container to ensure sterilization. Turn off the heat, and immediately pour the water onto the plant material. Add some salt—except to seaweed gargle, which contains its own.[2] Cover and steep. Gargle with as hot a tea as you can manage.

Gargle two to three times a day. Use about a quarter of a cup at a time. Store the remainder in the refrigerator, leaving the plant material inside to gather strength. The plant material will settle to the bottom. Pour off the amount of liquid needed, and reheat as necessary.

Josephine recommends seaweed, with its many minerals, as the best gargle, especially for tonsillitis.[3] For details on gathering, drying, processing, and storing seaweed, see the section on seaweed under Native Plant Foods.

While she was growing up, Josephine's family chewed pine pitch for sore throats. Sometimes company would bring them one or two seaweed cakes, but these didn't last long: *We'd just eat that down* [laughs]. *It gets moist and slips around in your mouth.*

To prevent gum problems, Josephine's Grandpa John had the children chew charcoal periodically: *We always got a big chunk of charcoal out of the heater stove, and then we'd crunch them up. That's how they purify water.*

Josephine learned about seaweed for gargles, and food, when she lived in Trinidad: *A lot of the old people on the coast used it. They even take it partly dry, heat bacon grease in a fry pan, just enough to crisp it up, and eat it.*

Inhalants

In her front room, Josephine has a wood-burning heater stove that she acquired with herb making in mind. To prevent colds and flu she keeps the wintertime air in her home moist by heating water and peppernut leaves atop her stove in an old Pyrex pot. Alternatively, she uses mint leaves of any available species, including peppermint, spearmint, lemon mint (citronella), and apple mint, although the latter, unlike the others, won't grow at low elevations. Whatever the selected herb, Josephine never uses more than one species at a time.

Rinses for Hair

For softening hair, boil a quart of water on the stove, then turn off the heat. Immediately pour the water over the whole top of a black (five-finger) fern or maidenhair fern, above where it flares. Steep, covered, until the rinse becomes a dark color, much stronger than a standard tea. Work into the hair for five minutes after shampooing so hair becomes soft.

To cleanse hair of lice, make a fresh gallon each time, using half as much wormwood leaves and their stems as water. Bring water to a boil, then turn off the heat.

Pour immediately over the leaves; it's not necessary to strain them out. Work the liquid, while still warm,[4] vigorously into the hair for about five minutes with about a teaspoon of shampoo so it will foam (The shampoo is a substitute for the Fels Naptha soap of Josephine's childhood). Let the hair half dry, then repeat the treatment. Let the hair dry for another thirty minutes or so, then rinse it with warm water. Wait two days, then repeat the entire process. This will usually be enough to rid the hair of lice, but if it isn't, wait three days and reapply. The wait between treatments gives the eggs time to hatch. Josephine adds: *Camphorated oil is another one that will kill lice. Just rub it in directly. You generally leave it on longer. That smell will stay in there for two or three days.*

Soaks

Josephine recommends using soaks to treat swelling from sprains, bruises, star thistle "*poisoning,*" skin diseases like psoriasis, arthritis, posterior yeast infections, rashes, and diabetic feet. Use enamel pots or basins. The pot or basin must be of sufficient size to allow for full coverage of the affected parts. Alternately, Josephine recommends the use of a bubble spa to aid circulation in swollen feet and legs. Use the spa without bubbles to keep the soak warm.

Boil water on the stove to sterilize it. Turn off the heat and pour the water immediately onto the herbs. If necessary, to cool the soak down to a comfortable temperature, add cold water. Josephine estimates that she uses a handful of herbs to a quart of water. While she doesn't measure the herbs, the stronger the decoction is, the more effective the soak. Before soaking, she pulls or strains out the herbs.

Soak the affected areas three to four times a day for at least half an hour. As a general rule, soak whenever the affected part becomes bothersome or burns. Continue soaking until the solution cools. Reheat as needed for additional later soaks.

When Josephine was growing up, people soaked in galvanized metal tubs. Her mother sometimes used five gallon cans of lard with the lid removed. Alternatively, she scrubbed out kerosene cans: *We always had those big, high cans a long time ago. We used to use old, square kerosene cans. We used to get kerosene in five gallon cans, and my mom would cut the top off and wash them out for soaking your legs.*

Josephine's father worked with cement, which caused boils and carbuncles to develop. He soaked his hands in Epsom salts in worn-out enamel canning pots, the white-speckled kind that Josephine refers to as granite: *We'd save them, and dad would plug them with cloth, because we couldn't use them for cooking fruit.* Whenever the water needed reheating, the pot was placed on the family's narrow potbellied heater stove. The plugged holes could be positioned off the stovetop.

Washes

Josephine primarily uses washes for treating yeast infections, diabetic sores, and athlete's foot. They may also be used for treating skin infections, rashes, including poison oak rash and itch, and sterilizing (cleansing) the area around sores.

Josephine estimates that she uses a handful of herbs to a quart of water. While Josephine doesn't measure the herbs, in general (as for soaks), the stronger the decoction is, the more effective the wash.

Boil the herbs directly in the water. Apply when comfortably warm. Keep applying until the wash cools. Repeat two to three more times a day, then apply a salve if needed. For poison oak, wash several times a day. With yeast infections, also wash several times a day, *whenever it gets to burning.*

Prepare eyewashes in the same manner and to the same strength as astandard tea. Use about three times a day. For cataracts, apply once a day for two days. Josephine also uses eyewashes on an occasional basis to relieve the strain on her eyes that develops from beading. When her favorite eyewash, acorn-leaching water, is unavailable, and the weather precludes an outing to gather herbs, she uses a light solution of boric acid. Acorn-leaching water will keep for about a month in the refrigerator.

Capsules

In recent years Josephine began using a mini-food mill to grind those dried herbs that taste bitter when brewed, then placing them in capsules, some ought-sized, some double ought, about half to three quarters of an inch in length. As Josephine explained: *We had no way to grind it way back. I started to use the capsules when I started getting cancer and AIDS patients. If they're going to make teas, they're going to do it for just a few days, and then they give it up. With a capsule, they'll keep taking it.*

Children have a hard time taking capsules, so Josephine reserves capsules for adults. Josephine uses the larger double ought capsules, about an inch in length, for blood purifiers, such as powdered Oregon grape and goldenseal. The latter, although bitter, is an effective liver cleanser. Grindelia, another good purifier, remains sticky even when dried, and can't be crushed up.

Poultices

Josephine recalls her mother making poultices to treat boils and carbuncles for her father with some type of bar soap, raw bacon, and a raw potato. Her mother also heated the bottom of a glass bottle in hot water, then held it with gloves or potholders over the boil. The unheated bottle neck was face down, against the skin: *Somehow it will suck it* [the core] *out.* Alternatively, a thread was twirled over the red core until it came out.

Josephine uses both fresh and dried herbs in her own poultices, except for those herbs that can't be mashed once dried, like spikenard root, which she only uses fresh. Before applying dried herbs, she steeps them in boiled water to activate the medicine and keep them in place when applied. She pours the boiling water onto the herbs immediately, without letting it cool, unlike with teas, where she lets the boiled water sit for three or four minutes before pouring it onto the herbs.

Josephine wraps the herbs with flannel or other soft cotton cloth to hold them in place. She has even used gauze, which holds the plant material well. A long time ago, it was necessary to apply a hot wash rag or hot water bottle atop poultices to keep them moist. Heat generates sweat, which opens the pores, so the herbs can penetrate the skin. *We even used to heat rocks from the river bar on our heater stoves.* These smooth, flat rocks were wrapped in a towel and put into the children's beds to warm them. After walking home from school in the rain, the children could warm up this way. If they sprained an ankle, heat also helped.

Josephine neither knots nor tucks in the cloth. Rather, she covers her poultices with Saran plastic wrap to retain the moisture, and advises her patients to keep the affected part still. For victims of stroke and blood poisoning, Josephine suggests keeping the poultice on continuously, including at night. Whenever a poultice needs to be reapplied, always make it with new herbs. For those patients who can stay at home, Josephine suggests they consider using soaks instead of poultices.

Josephine has never seen anyone have an allergic reaction to poultices, which, since they're applied externally, can be easily monitored to gauge their effect. Josephine recalls one incident when a woman digging spikenard root in a gully mistakenly dug the roots of a nearby poison oak plant. Later, the woman broke out in a rash. To prevent the rash after exposure to poison oak, Josephine recommends thoroughly rinsing the affected skin with soda water.

Pastes

Reducing an herb to a paste-like consistency enables it to be spread smoothly. Josephine recommends adding a little olive oil to some herbs, boiled water to others. In limited instances fresh leaves or root may be mashed, then poulticed, rather than creating a paste.

For chest colds, Josephine makes a thick, nighttime poultice from mustard flowers, or mustard powder mixed with flour and an egg. For details, see "Mustard, yellow." For treating diabetic sores, Josephine prefers a peppernut plaster, due to its ability to draw. Before poulticing, she runs dried peppernuts through a food mill, then adds enough olive oil to hold the particles together.

Plasters

Plasters are poulticed pastes, created by smoothing a paste onto a soft cloth. To prevent skin blisters, Josephine applies a layer of cloth between the skin and plastered paste.

Salves

As a child, Josephine used to prepare salves in a white, granite pot with her paternal grandmother. Although she no longer remembers the recipes, she recalls that her "*old grandmas*" used to use white clover. Since then, she has developed her own recipes.

Josephine makes salves after the first full moon in April, when the plants are at their optimum. If gathered any earlier than this, the leaves won't be big enough. The flower will sometimes pull the strength out of a plant, so Josephine prefers harvesting before the flowers bud. When using flowers, she prefers fresh blossoms, but substitutes dried flowers when fresh ones aren't available. With some plants, the blossoms shrivel immediately upon harvest, so there isn't any choice. When using the upper part of a plant, Josephine generally uses the leaves and blossoms, setting the stem aside. Although the stem can be included, leaves and flowers alone are easier to strain out. She washes the roots and cuts them into pieces of an inch or so. She tears the leaves apart so the veins are opened up, and the medicine can seep out.

Josephine stores dried salve-making plants—wild cherry bark, wormwood flower tips, yarrow leaves, and turkey mullein leaves—in a cardboard box, so that they may be used when fresh herbs aren't available.

Josephine uses only "*natural*" 100 percent pure virgin olive oil in her salves. Not only is this oil good for healing skin diseases in general, but, unlike other oils, it does

Figure 3.6.
Josephine *(right)* sharing salve
making with Zona Ferris and
Deborah E. McConnell. Photo by
LaVerne Glaze.

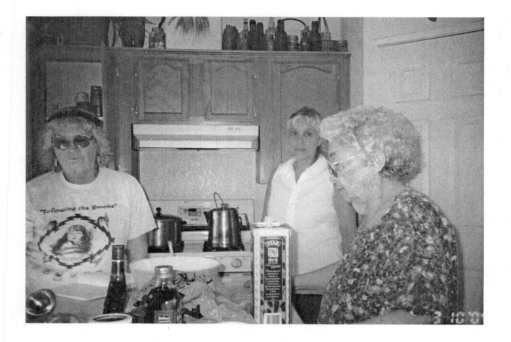

not contain preservatives. She heats the oil until it's good and hot (close to boiling) before adding the plant material, which the oil should cover. Josephine usually heats the oil in a Pyrex coffee pot on her woodstove, then removes the pot from direct heat by placing it on the back of the stove. Next, she adds the herbs, and leaves the mixture there to simmer overnight. (The herbs may also be added with the oil, then both heated together.) Every thirty minutes or so, she swirls the pot to mix its contents. Alternatively, stir the mixture every thirty minutes or so with a wooden spoon (never metal), so the plant soaks up the oil. Sometimes the plant material will float atop the oil, so stirring keeps it down.

Josephine recommends against simmering salves atop a modern stove, because regulating the heat is easier on a woodstove. When a woodstove isn't available, she mixes the herbs and oil together in a Pyrex bowl or pan, then heats them in an oven. She recommends setting the temperature at about 200 degrees so the oil won't boil. Every thirty minutes or so she shakes the bowl or pan around to keep the herbs mixed in.

Relative batch size is a factor in deciding whether to simmer or bake salves. Simmering on a stovetop works best for small batches (those with one pint of oil); baking in an oven is better for larger batches.

To strain out the herbs, Josephine rubber bands a piece of flour sack around the open top of a jar, loosely enough so the cloth dips down in the middle. Then she pours the simmered herb mixture atop the cloth. Josephine's grandmother used salt sacks, with their tight weave, or flour sacks, with their somewhat looser weave. Clean rags provide an apt substitute. She recommends against coffee filters, which oil won't easily penetrate. She also recommends against screen strainers, due to the possibility that the metal will contaminate the herbs, although sometimes screen strainers are the only thing available.

Josephine transfers the strained salve mixture into baby-food or other small jars, leaving enough room for the beeswax she adds next.[5] She places the jars in a pan

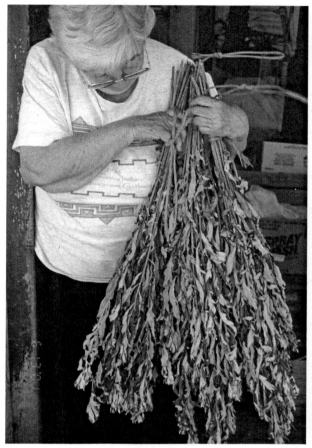

Figure 3.7.
Wormwood drying. Once dry, it will be broken apart and stored in a gallon jar to help it retain its "strength." When stored in paper bags herbs lose their strength within six months. Photo by Beverly Ortiz.

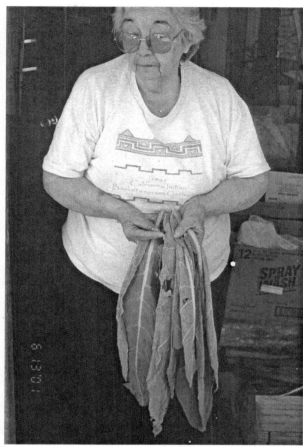

Figure 3.8.
Josephine Peters taking down dried mullein leaves in her Hoopa Valley porch. Photo by Beverly Ortiz.

of hot water on her heater stove, so the jars don't break, since the strained salve mixture is also hot when the jars are placed inside of it. While this water bath needs to be hot enough to melt the wax in the jars, it shouldn't be allowed to boil, or some of the strained salve mixture will boil out. The pan should be low, such as a frying pan or metal baking pan. Since the jar separates the medicine from the metal of the pan, there's no concern about contamination. The water should reach about three-quarters of the way up the jars.

When Josephine was growing up, her family had two bee hives. A canvas mask with a screen in front provided her father's only protection when working with bees. After removing a honey comb frame, he'd bring it to Josephine's mother, who placed it over a round enamel milk pan some four or five inches high and fifteen inches across.[6] After the honey dripped out, the children would take what remained of the comb and chew it up for a special treat.

Josephine learned how much beeswax to add to her salves by trial and error. If needed, she adds additional wax after the jars have been placed in the hot water bath. All told, she estimates that she chops off a teaspoon- to a tablespoon-sized piece per baby food jar. While the jars are in the water bath, she stirs the wax with a Popsicle stick or wooden skewer, the type used to stir coffee, until the wax melts into the medicine, which happens rather quickly, at times in about ten minutes. Stirring keeps the wax from floating to the top of the oil. To remove the hot jars from the water bath, Josephine uses a clamp for canning that fits around the top of each jar. A hot pad may also be used. She places the jars on a wooden "*meat board*," and continues stirring until the mixture cools and thickens. Once the jars are cold, she puts the lids on them. If the lids are added to soon, the salve will sweat inside the jar. Baby food jars will form a seal. Other jars will not, but a seal isn't necessary so long as the lid is twisted tight.

Alternatively, Josephine removes the entire water bath from the stove and places the pan on a wooden meat board. Continue stirring the salve until it cools and thickens. Place the lids on the jars.

Apply salves at least three or four times a day, including once in the morning and once before going to bed.

Salve Recipe for Treating Sunburn, Eczema, Poison Oak, Psoriasis, and Dry Skin, Such as On the Elbows [7]

Preheat oven to 250 degrees. Wash ten fresh leaves each of dandelion, wide-leaved plantain, ribbed plantain, and four leaves of mullein. To wash the leaves, hold them under the faucet. Tear the washed leaves into approximately one-inch pieces.

Put leaf pieces into a large ovenproof (Pyrex) glass bowl. [8] Pour two pints of Star olive oil over the leaves. Heat at 250 degrees for one hour. According to Josephine, this will reduce each pint of olive oil to the amount that will fill two baby food jars. A double batch, with two pints of oil, yields ten baby food jars. When making one pint, halve the plant material.

Strain the mixture [9] into a glass bowl or jar. Pour the strained oil into baby food jars [10] about two-thirds full, leaving enough room to add beeswax. Depending on their relative size, put two or three chunks of beeswax into each jar. Each chunk should be about the size of a quarter. Place jars in a shallow pan of water (hot water bath) on the stovetop, and heat to melt the wax, stirring continuously with a wooden skewer (non-metal; non-plastic). [11] The wax melts completely within one half to one hour. Add more wax as needed to get the right consistency (solid but soft when cooled). The salve will start to thicken on the edges of the jar—that helps you see when the consistency is about right. Remove the jars from the water bath, and continue to stir for a few more minutes so the salve won't separate while it cools. Once the salve is completely cooled, put lids on the jars.

Salve Recipe for Treating Ulcerated Sores, External Cancerous Sores, and Bedsores [12]

This salve recipe works especially well on bedsores, particularly for those patients who don't get up and move around. Thoroughly wash the roots and lower stems of fresh coltsfoot. [13] While holding the coltsfoot under running water, scrub it clean with an old toothbrush, then break off the fine side-roots. In the past, Josephine used a wooden brush with bristles for the purpose, the type used to brush and wash animals. Clean the root out-of-doors lest the dirt plug the plumbing. Cut about one handful of root into one-inch lengths.

Gather a handful of fresh Johnny-jump-ups, an aspirin-like pain reliever, and remove the roots. Washed roots may be included, and, when flowering, Johnny-

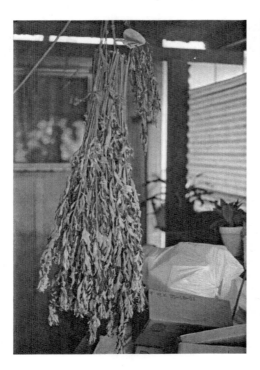

Figure 3.9.
Wormwood hung to dry in Josephine's porch.
Photo by Beverly Ortiz.

jump-up blossoms may be added. Gather, as well, a handful of fresh heal-all, including the roots. When flowering, heal-all blossoms may be added. Wash the violet and heal-all, then tear them into smaller pieces before adding.

Have a handful of fresh, or an equivalent amount of dried, mugwort flowers and their little stems at the ready. Josephine prefers to use the young tops of mugwort plants that have grown about six inches high and haven't yet blossomed. However, it's okay to substitute older plant tops, including the stem and flowers, but never the roots. Mugwort flowers in late summer. When dry, the plant isn't as strong, so Josephine uses somewhat more than when fresh.

Cut beeswax into chunks about the size of a quarter. Not all the chunks will end up the same size.

Put the coltsfoot, violet, heal-all, and one pint of olive oil into a Pyrex coffee pot. Heat slowly for about thirty minutes, until the mixture nearly boils, then turn down the heat, stir with a wooden spoon (non-metal; non-plastic), and add the dried mugwort flowers.[14] Heat gently for a short time longer, then turn off the heat and let the mixture cool a bit. Josephine prefers to let the mixture cool overnight on the back of her heater stove.

Strain the mixture[15] into a glass bowl or jar. Pour the strained oil into baby food jars until they're about two-thirds full, leaving enough room to add beeswax. Depending on their relative size, put two or three chunks of beeswax into each jar. Place jars in a shallow pan of water on the stovetop and heat to melt the wax, stirring continuously with a wooden skewer or flat stick.[16] Add more wax as needed to get the right consistency—solid but soft when cooled. It will take about fifteen minutes for the wax to melt. The salve will start to thicken on the edges of the jar—that helps you see when the consistency is about right. Remove the jars from the water bath, and continue to stir for a few more minutes so the salve won't separate while it cools. Once cold, put lids on the jars.

Salve Recipe for Treating Impetigo, Infected Sores, and Ulcerated Sores[17]

Put olive oil in a Pyrex coffee pot and *heat it up good on the stove*. Add an equal amount of plantain leaves (wide-leaf or narrow) and dandelion (washed root, stem, and leaves in the summertime; washed root in the wintertime), and one large leaf of mullein.[18] As for the amount of dandelion and plantain leaves to add, like all experienced cooks, Josephine doesn't measure: *I just throw a bunch together. Just let it sit in there, and simmer it down...so it will get all the good out of the plants... Then you put the wax in, and mix it up good while it's hot. Just simmer it. Some of it gets nice and spongy.* (For a recipe using these same plants to make a salve for skin diseases, see above.)

Alternative Salve Recipe for Treating Infected and Ulcerated Sores[19]

This recipe may be used to treat impetigo, but is ineffective for this disease unless it absorbs beneath the outer skin. Unlike the other salves, it should not be used for sores if the patient has scratched their skin raw.

Use the three, pitchy *brown things* on the tips of cottonwood branches when they come out in the spring (February or March). Combine a heaping teaspoon of cottonwood tips, five leaves of ribbed plantain and mullein leaves. Use one heaping teaspoon of cottonwood tips, five leaves of ribbed plantain, and a single, big leaf of mullein some eight to ten inches long. Double the amount to make more. Follow the general salve-making recipe above.

Mullein is an especially good herb for treating sores that don't heal, although this varies according to type of sore and the medicine used. Peppernut poultices are especially beneficial for diabetic sores, for instance; coltsfoot poultices for miners who got sores from wearing gumboots all the time.

Salve Recipe for Treating Boils, Ulcerated Sores, and Skin Diseases, like Psoriasis, Scabies, Mange on Animals, and Ringworm[20]

Use coltsfoot root, plantain leaf, and wormwood leaves. If there's pain, add a little garden violet (see Johnny-jump-up) to kill it. For a quart of salve, use about five, four-inch-long roots of coltsfoot, about eight leaves of plantain (wide-leaf or narrow, aka ribbed), a *good handful* of crushed wormwood leaves, and about five or six whole Johnny-jump-up plants, including the roots. Wash the roots before adding. Tear the plants into smaller pieces to release the medicine. Follow the recipe for open sores above. In the case of boils, first remove the core before applying the salve. See "Poultices" for methods to remove it.

Cough Syrups

At the Old Home Place, the family's contemporary name for the ranch where Josephine grew up, there were few store-bought remedies. Castoria served as a laxative. Josephine's mother made cough syrup for colds from a chopped onion steamed or simmered in a china bowl on the back of the family's woodstove: *She must have put sugar in it, because it was sweet. I'd try it, but never did use it in my own doctoring.*

Josephine makes syrups year round, usually with mountain balm and horehound. She adds roughly the same amount of the leaves and stem of each. She uses mountain balm, an evergreen, fresh; she sometimes dries horehound and cuts it up in a chopper, and in this case uses a lot less than if it were fresh. Mints, another component, work well dried. In fact, in syrups Josephine uses more dried than fresh herbs.

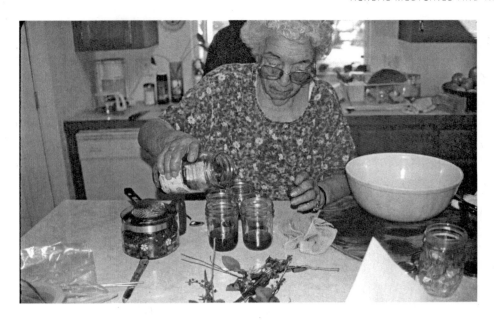

Figure 3.10.
Josephine Peters transferring the strained cough syrup mixture into jars. Photo by Deborah E. McConnell.

Josephine prescribes syrups to people of all ages (unlike cough drops, see below). Small babies get about three drops from a dropper diluted in some water. Babies of about a year-and-a-half to a year can take about half a teaspoon to a full teaspoon; children of about eight two teaspoons. At nine years and up, they can begin to take the adult dosage of about two tablespoons.

Nowadays, Josephine makes two gallons of cough syrup at a time. As she explains, *When that flu hits, everybody comes. I give them a quart.*

To make cough syrup, put water and fresh or dried herbs together in a Pyrex coffee pot. The water usually covers the plants, but less can be added if you want thicker syrup. For eight ounces of syrup, Josephine estimates that she uses about six ounces of water, a good heaping tablespoon of dried horehound leaves, and five or six whole, big leaves of mountain balm.

Josephine heats the hot water and herbs in a Pyrex pot until the water nearly boils, then she simmers them: *Let it simmer until it goes way down. When you let it evaporate on the back of a* [wood-burning] *stove, it'll get down to where you don't have that much left.* Strain the mixture with a flour sack, then add just under two ounces of honey while the water is still hot, shaking to mix it in: *The honey will help thicken it. But you can't get it too thick either, because it'll be hard to swallow. You don't want it to really set hard.* Once the mixture has cooled, add two teaspoons of brandy as a preservative, or rum when brandy isn't available. Use a good quality brandy, such as Original Extra Smooth E & J., eighty proof, forty percent alcohol by volume. Finally, transfer the syrup into six- to eight-ounce bottles, which Josephine prefers over jars. Once cold, seal the bottles.

For treating asthma and whooping cough, Josephine adds half-inch-long marijuana buds to her syrups: *[T]hat calms them. It keeps them from coughing. People bring me the buds to use.* One bud will suffice for a small amount: *You don't put much, just enough to stop the spasm.* For children, Josephine uses an amount approximating the size of half a dime. For adults, she adds about two or three buds to her standard recipe. Josephine adds: *If you look at any kind of cough medicine, it's got hemp in it.* Alternatively, add six marijuana seeds in place of a half inch bud.

The seeds are more potent than the buds. When buds aren't available, Josephine sometimes adds shake.[21]

Babies exposed to drugs in the womb are susceptible to lung problems. As with asthma, they have difficulty breathing, often coughing until they nearly lose their breath. Such babies need close watching. To treat their symptoms, Josephine mixes orange juice with a little honey and a tiny bit of marijuana. She gives them about three quarters of a teaspoon.

Syrup Recipe for Cough, Asthma, Bronchitis, Whooping Cough, and Pneumonia [22]

Place one to two good handfuls each of wild choke-cherry bark (gathered in the fall and dried), the tops of fresh heal-all, and fresh mountain balm leaves in a Pyrex pot. There's no set amount of herbs to add; rather, it's up to the discretion of the cook, based on her experience. You can tear up the leaves to release the medicine.

Add just enough cold water to cover the plants. Bring almost to a boil, then stir with a wooden spoon and push the plants down to the bottom. Lower the heat and continue simmering for about thirty minutes. Turn off the heat. Add one or two handfuls of wormwood flowers, about four inflorescence stems some four inches long covered in flowers, and stir.

For asthma, bronchitis, whooping cough and pneumonia, add one tablespoon of marijuana shake. Alternatively, add one tablespoon marijuana seeds, or enough marijuana bud to stop the coughing spasms. A partial bud is enough, a quarter inch for a child.

To remove all of the sediment, strain out the herbs into a glass jar, in this case with an available open weave basket covered with flour sacking. Add one pint of honey and swirl the jar to mix it in well. Add one quarter cup of brandy while the syrup is still warm.

Pour into any available, clean jars—mayonnaise and jam jars, for instance. Let cool, then put the lids on. Keep syrup in the refrigerator. Take one tablespoon several times a day to suppress coughs. Make the syrup half-strength for a child. Give a baby a dilute form with a dropper.

Syrup Recipe for Cough [23]

Place a good handful each of the fresh stem and leaves of horehound and mountain balm into a Pyrex pot. To make a pint of syrup, use about seven or eight fresh leaves of mountain balm, the amount of leaves that can be crushed in one's fist. Add an equal amount, or a little less, of horehound. If the leaves are dry, run them through a chopper and add about one heaping tablespoonful. For cooking instructions, follow the previous recipe. Use only brandy, not rum, in this syrup.

Syrup Recipe for Asthma and Whooping Cough [24]

For adults, add a few marijuana buds to the mountain balm and horehound cough syrup described above, in the same ratios as the other syrup recipes.

Cough Drops

At the Old Home Place, when Josephine and her siblings got a sore throat, they'd gather pine pitch and chew it. Their parents also bought horehound candy for the children. Today, Josephine generally reserves cough drops for adults, lest children accidentally swallow or choke on them. The youngest patients to whom she dispenses cough drops are seven or eight, but, even then, she prefers that children take syrup. When syrup is unavailable, Josephine breaks a drop in half for them to take. By the time they're twelve, they can take a whole drop.

To make the drops, put somewhat more honey than water in a Pyrex pot. Use the equivalent of about three quarters of a cup of honey to half a cup water. Heat this, then pour the mixture over the prescribed herbs. While Josephine prefers honey, brown sugar may be substituted in a ratio of about a quarter of a cup to one cup of water.

Add ten to twelve leaves of horehound to every pint. If using dried leaves, crush the horehound in a blender or chopper, and add one tablespoonful. Alternatively, use half this amount each of horehound and mountain balm. You can also use mountain balm exclusively, but Josephine prefers to mix the two.

Simmer the mixture until it reaches a light boil, strain it, and return what remains to the pot. Put the pot on the back of the heater stove to evaporate the drops down slowly, or, to make them quickly, simmer until finished on a source of direct heat.

The drops are ready if, when you dip a spoon into the mixture, a little *hair* comes off it. They're not ready if the mixture drips off the spoon quickly. As an alternative method of testing the mixture's readiness, drop a little bit into cold water. If it forms a hard ball, it's done.

To mold her drops, Josephine pours the mixture into a glass container that once held Chinese medicine or candy. Reminiscent of an egg carton, it has sixteen marble-sized holes. If such a container isn't available, pour the mixture onto wax paper, as in making peanut brittle, then chop it into cough-drop sized pieces. Let it set (harden) all day.

NATIVE PLANT FOODS

Fruit

As a child, Josephine, the oldest girl in her family, used to go out on her own and pick fruit—blackberries, blackcaps, domestic red raspberries, gooseberries, huckleberries, thimbleberries, and wild strawberries, all uncultivated; and loganberries and youngberries, planted by her mother in two rows of each. Elderberries did not grow at *the ranch*, or *Old Home*, although there were *plenty around* in other areas. Josephine eschewed elderberries, however, due to their taste, which she considered *kind of funny*. Blueberries could be obtained and eaten off the bush at higher elevations, but there weren't enough to cook with.

As Josephine got older, her siblings joined in gathering *berries: We'd eat all the best ones [laughs] while picking them. There was a campground across the river... I'd take it over and sell them... We had the old-fashioned kind of blackberries that grew all over in the old mine. It had a different shape and leaf* [than those growing in the Hoopa Valley today]. The old mine was a ponded area on the Old Home Place that had resulted from hydraulic mining. Its berries were long, not round in shape. Their leaves were two to three inches across. Josephine sold blackberries, which ripened in July and August, for about three dollars per gallon.

Josephine recommends that the relatively *mushy* fruit of thimbleberries and salmonberries, and the tiny fruit of wild strawberries, always be eaten raw. The fruit of elderberries must be cooked, since, when eaten raw, this fruit can make a person feel sick.

Josephine gathers berries into small containers, usually pots and pans, so they won't get crushed. The Old Home Place was situated far enough from roads that the berries weren't exposed to dust. Today, those that grow near roads must be rinsed: *You've got to wash them right away, as soon as you get them home, because they juice up really bad.* Place the berries in a colander, run water over them, and let them drip overnight. Josephine freezes some berries for later use in cottage cheese and yogurt containers. She also uses freezer bags.

Gooseberries

As a child, Josephine use to lay a gunny sack beneath a gooseberry bush, then would beat the berries off with a stick. She would roll a handful of berries between any two handy, flat rocks in a counterclockwise direction. This knocked off the "*stickers*" without damaging the skin. She popped what remained between her teeth. She brought those she didn't eat home, or sold them to tourists in the campground across the river.

For gooseberry pie with a flour crust, Josephine's maternal grandmother put the berries in a flat pan on the kitchen table. She used a rolling pin to open them up and release the juice, then thickened the juice with cornstarch until it was pudding-like: *When it gets cold, it's really firm.* See "Pies" for a crust recipe.

Huckleberries

Josephine gathers huckleberries off fire roads, where they're clean. Once home, she winnows the berries in a basket to remove any plant debris. On windy days, she sometimes uses two baskets, pouring the berries from one basket into the other. To dry the berries, Josephine places them in the sun in a winnowing basket on her porch steps. She places a stiff, mesh cloth over the top of the berries to protect them from animals and insects. At night, she takes the basket and berries inside her home, lest her pets sleep on them. Once dried, Josephine uses huckleberries for pie: *Boil it good and add thickening.*

Manzanita Berries

A lot of manzanita bushes grew at *the ranch*, or *Old Home*, where Josephine grew up. Later in life, Josephine gathered manzanita berries from bushes growing off fire roads, where the berries are clean: *We go up in the mountains and pick, if we can beat the bears to them* [laughs]. Pick large clumps of the red, ripe berries by the handful. Remove the stems by rolling the berries in a circular, open-work basket woven close enough to contain the fruit, but open enough for the stems to fall through.

Josephine's mother made a sweet drink from manzanita berries by pounding the red, ripened berries in a wooden bowl until the skin powdered: *Of course they've got a lot of seed in them, and not much powder. She'd pound it all up, and put it in a gallon jar. She used to call it cider. It made a nice drink... We'd drink it like we do Kool Aid.* Josephine loved manzanita cider as a child.

The sweetness leached from the powder as it sat in cold water in the jar. Once the water was sweet, Josephine's mother strained out the powder through a flour sack.

Josephine powders her berries by putting them through the biggest chopper in an old meat grinder. She sifts out the hard seeds, some of which get broken up, with a screen sifter or handled sieve. She soaks the powder in a big jar, stirring it up before drinking.

Cooking with Fruit

Canned Fruit

Josephine learned to can as a child. Today, canning is still commonly practiced in the Hoopa Valley, although less so among the young and those without families. Josephine cans native blackberries, non-Native Himalaya berries, and huckleberries. Neighbors and friends also share cultivated fruit with each other, lest it spoil. One week a crop of peaches may arrive, another, plums, and, the next, a box of tomatoes. Josephine's mother canned in two-quart jars. As Josephine explained with a laugh: *We had a big family. There were eleven of us, and there were always some others around.*

To can fruit, first fill the jar with fruit. Then: *Put a little sugar, but not too much. I always mark the* [jars] *I make pie out of. I don't put sugar in them at all, because then you might put more sugar in and make it too sweet... * [I] *seal them and put them in a* [hot] *water bath for twenty-five minutes. When they're sealed, they stay sealed. A lot of people take the rings off, and you can hear them pop open when it gets hot. I keep the rings on them.*

Jams and Jellies

Jelly sets firm; jam doesn't: *We never paid for jam and jelly then. We went out ourselves and got* [gathered] *what we wanted.* For jam, Josephine prefers blackberries, since these have relatively few seeds. The non-native cherry plum, cultivated in the Hoopa Valley for its yellow to orange fruits, was also used by locals for jam, although Josephine, who made it once, did not like its strong, acidy flavor.

For jelly, Josephine uses loganberries and youngberries, both non-native species that were planted in profusion at the Old Home Place: *We had a couple of rows of each of those.* Occasionally, Josephine makes both jam and jelly with huckleberries, but always in equal proportion to blackberries: *They're tiny and it takes so long to clean them, I mix* [huckleberries] *with some other kind of juice.*
When Josephine can obtain enough native blackcaps, she also uses these to make jam and jelly: *Blackcaps generally come up where there's been an old burn... Blackcaps are like raspberries, but dark. One old man would pick them and bring them to me.*

Today, blackcaps, used for jellies and and jams throughout Josephine's childhood, have become hard to find. Josephine finds the plants growing in areas logged off two or three years before, but the birds and bears usually eat them first. In addition to berries, Maggie Bennett Grant made apple and plum jellies and jams.

Josephine prepares her jams and jellies in the same basic manner, except that for jam, she retains the pulp, rather than straining it. After gathering her berries, Josephine rinses them as soon as she can. Next, she cooks down the berries, until they come apart, then strains those intended for jelly though an old flour sack, with its relatively loose weave. As Josephine explains about loganberries and youngberries: *They have little tiny seeds. Always cook them, then let them sit overnight and strain them, so you don't get seeds.* To complete her jams and jellies, Josephine adds sugar in equal proportions to the pulp or juice, then cooks this down until it thickens. It's done when it slips, as a jelled unit, from a spoon.

Maggie used an enamel milk pan to cook her berries. Josephine has cooked hers in an enamel roaster at 300 degrees. Moisture evaporates out of the berries more slowly in the oven, so that they thicken gradually. When boiled atop the stove, the berries can scorch. Josephine prefers this method, however, since it's faster. To avoid scorching, she keeps the flame relatively low.

Once the berries are cooked, she puts them in jars, adds wax, and places the jars in a water bath. For her water bath, Josephine uses a pot about eight inches across, lower than the tops of the jars, and big enough to hold four: *We just leave it in there until the wax melts, and take it out. It gets pretty hot in there. We don't let it boil. Always turn it down just below boiling.*

Pastry

Duff

Josephine makes duff with blackberries, huckleberries, or apples. Clean the berries. Simmer them with cornstarch to thicken the mixture. Add a little cinnamon and sugar.

Make a biscuit dough, sweetened with sugar, using baking powder instead of yeast. Blend three quarter cups of sugar, two eggs, one tablespoon of baking powder, and a half cup of shortening, then add two cups of flour. When using butter, add a whole cube (one-half cup).

Drop dough teaspoonful by teaspoonful into the thickened berries, and let the mixture cook. When Josephine was growing up, duff was made in enamel containers. Today she uses a 10 x 15 inch Pyrex baking dish.

At the September 23, 2001, wedding of the daughter of one of Josephine's foster children, a variation of duff was served. The dough was laid atop the thickened berries, which were placed in a flat, metal baking pan.

Pie

Make pie with any locally available, clean, fleshy berries. Josephine makes pies with fresh blackberries in the summertime, and apples, peaches and cherries when they ripen on the trees in her yard. For her crusts, Josephine uses shortening or lard, flour and water in "*one-two-three*" proportions: one cup shortening, two cups flour, and three tablespoons water. If the crust doesn't feel right, add a little more water, taking care not to add too much.[25] A pinch of salt may also be added. About shortening, Josephine says: *Bear fat makes the best pie crust because it's oily... Chop it up small and put it in the oven to render.*

Place the berries in the crust, and sprinkle them with a mixture of flour, sugar, and spices (mostly cinnamon, sometimes nutmeg). When using a graham cracker crust, thicken the berries on top of the stove with cornstarch or flour. When this becomes pudding like, pour it in the crust. Serve with fresh cream.

Fried Pies

Josephine's Aunt Mary made fried pies with apples, berries, lemons, even store-bought canned pineapple. Josephine recommends blackberries, blackcaps, domestic raspberries, huckleberries, and domestic strawberries. Other berries have too many seeds, or are too tiny or mushy. To make a fried pie, cut a circle of dough around a desert plate (see pies, above, for ingredients). Form a crescent shape by folding the circle of dough in half. Press the edges together to seal all but an opening large enough to fit a tablespoon. Cook the fruit with cornstarch to thicken it, then spoon the mixture into the dough: *We'd fill that little tart up, then press it down good so it would be sealed, and cook it in oil* [like a donut]. *That was good.*

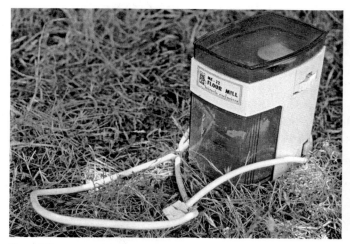

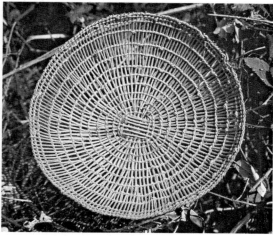

Figure 3.11.
Flour mill used by Josephine today for processing acorns. Photo by
Beverly Ortiz.

Figure 3.12.
Basket used by Josephine Peters for leaching. A porous cotton
cloth is laid atop the basket prior to leaching. Photo by Beverly
Ortiz, 2009.

Josephine's mother made her fried pies with shortening; today Josephine uses
vegetable oil. When available, use rendered bear fat to deep fry donuts and fried pie.

Steam Pudding

Maggie Bennett Grant made steam pudding, which Josephine describes as bread-
like. Make a biscuit dough, as you would for duff (see above).

Add raisins or huckleberries, and form the dough into a ball. Wrap it in cheese-
cloth, place it in a double boiler, and steam until cooked. Remove the cloth. Make a
sauce from water, vinegar, thickener (cornstarch), nutmeg and a little cinnamon to
taste. Josephine adds: *We used to have a lot of butter, and sometimes mom would
drop about a tablespoon of it into the sauce to make it taste good. We'd pour that
sauce over it and eat it. It was really good.* Slice the "*pudding.*"

Mushrooms

Canned Mushrooms

Clean tanoak, chanterelle, or commercial mushrooms. Add boiling water to mushrooms in a canning jar. Seal the lid, then boil for thirty minutes. Fish and meat need
to be boiled for ninety minutes.

Venison and Tanoak Mushroom Casserole

Chop the venison into inch squares, add flour, and brown in lard: *A long time ago
everything was lard.* Add two tablespoons of chopped onion, and salt and pepper to
taste. Simmer until the meat is tender. Add two cups of acorn soup and one cup of
finely chopped mushrooms, then simmer for another fifteen minutes until the mushrooms cook. Remove from heat and transfer into a flat baking dish. Make a biscuit-
like dough, patting it out on a cutting board about an inch in thickness, enough
to cover the entire dish. Bake at 350 degrees and cook until the bread is done. *We
always made this in the fall, during the hunting season, when the mushrooms were
out. It was like us having a thanksgiving* [laughs].

Nuts

Acorns

A "*good crop*" of acorn occurs every fourth year, so Josephine gathers more than a year's supply: *We always use tanoak when it's plentiful.* Once or twice, Josephine has gathered the long, slender acorns of white oak near Redding.

Dry acorns in a box near the woodstove for a month or so. If gathered before the rains, they'll already be somewhat dry, and can be laid rather thickly in the box. Turn the nuts once or twice daily, whenever you think about it, so that the acorns in the middle don't mold.

Crack the nuts with a hammer, butt-end up. If you crack the nuts while they're fresh, they turn an unsightly gray color due to bruising. When dry, the nuts virtually pop out of the shell.

Use last year's nuts with a few of the fresh to *boost up the taste*. With tanoak, the skin comes right off, so there's no need to winnow. With white oak, the skin stays on: *You have to break it off.*

Run the nuts through a Miracle Flour Mill, using the smallest gauge, so the flour will be as fine as possible. When fine, the flour will "*soak*" (leach) in a couple of hours. When the flour has big chunks, it takes longer to soak.

Josephine uses two twined baskets for leaching, a relatively finely woven basket made by Madelaine Davis, and a round-bottomed one woven by "Honey Bunch" Perry. She places a cloth atop the basket, and the acorn flour atop this, as much as an inch-and-a-half deep depending on the amount of acorn to be leached. The cloth must be "*soft*" (relatively porous), or water won't leach through it. Josephine uses an old flour sack or flannel. A sheet isn't soft enough.

If making an eyewash, place the basket atop a bowl in the kitchen sink. Adjust the faucet water temperature until it's tepid, and let it drip through the acorn, filling the bowl. Stir, to get the flour all watery and break up the bumps. If not saving the water, prop the basket on a colander.

Drip tepid water through the flour for about two hours. This process removes a yellowish-colored oil and speeds up the leaching process. If only cold water were used, leaching would take all day.

In place of a water break, Josephine changes the position of her faucet from time to time, so the flour will leach evenly. If, after about two hours, the flour isn't fully leached, Josephine switches from tepid water to cold. She lets the cold water drip onto the acorn flour until not a hint of bitterness (tannin) remains: *People who leave the bitterness in turn others against ever eating it. I always take all mine out.*

Cook in a stainless steel pot, stirring with a big wooden spoon lest the acorn be burned on the bottom. Never use aluminum, as acorn will react with the metal. One cup of acorns will make a quart of mush. The cooked "*acorn soup*" should have a "*pretty thick*," mush-like consistency. When people prefer it thinner, they can always add water to it.

Josephine learned acorn making when she lived in Trinidad. She and an "*old lady*," an elder Yurok woman, would go up to a place along the coast near Gold Bluff where a high bank with an indentation was located, and water dripped off the mountain. The woman created a sand-leaching basin there, sometimes covered with coltsfoot or maple leaves, sometimes not. Maple leaf was available seasonally, whereas coltsfoot's large leaves are perennial. The woman used a V-shaped board trough to direct the water onto her acorn flour. As the acorn leached throughout the day, she and Josephine wove baskets.

After leaching was complete, the woman diverted the trough, so the water no longer dripped onto the flour. As the flour dried, it became caked enough to stick to her hand: *Then you can turn it upside down in your hand and wash the sand off.*

Josephine learned about white oak from Flora Jones (Wintun). At the State Indian Museum's annual Acorn Festival, they serve soup made from valley oak, a long acorn that turns purplish-looking when it's fixed, perhaps from chlorine in the water. At Morongo, the Cahuilla have "*little, bitty*" acorns about a half to three-quarters of an inch long. Josephine uses these sweet-tasting acorns, which don't require any leaching, for earrings. When the caps fall off, she puts a loop through them, then glues the caps back on. Inspired by acorn necklaces made by Robinson Pomo women, Josephine does the same with the larger valley oak (*Quercus lobata*) in the Ukiah area.

Acorn Biscuits and Bread.

I make a lot of acorn biscuits. When the hunters go out [they] can put two or three in their pockets and go. When they eat it, then drink water, it swells in their stomach and fills them up. Leach acorn in the sink as described above, retaining the first batch of water that leaches through as an eyewash to reduce cataracts. Leave the acorn there until it dries out. Place one cupful at a time of leached and dried acorn on a cookie sheet. Bake slowly in the oven. The resulting "*biscuits*" will be about an inch and a half or so in diameter.

For acorn bread, let the "acorn soup" dry after cooking. The water will come to the top. Pour off the water, then bake the remainder slowly in the oven. *See also:* peppernuts, below.

Hazelnuts

Hazelnuts look like large filberts. Gather them in the fall: *We used to go out and pick a big bucketful.* The husk, or covering, that encases the nut, with its hard shell, has a kind of fuzz of brownish hairs that stick up from the top. Care must be taken to grab the fuzz and peel it off: *That fuzz'll get on your fingers, and you'll just itch.* When I asked Josephine if the taste was worth the itch, she said: *Oh, yes. We didn't mind when we were kids!* Whenever the fuzz got in one's fingers, it could be washed off with water from a nearby river, creek, ditch, or pond. Today, Josephine recommends that rubber gloves be worn when husking the nuts. Dry them, as you would fresh walnuts. To shell them, Josephine and her family members used a rock or hammer.

Peppernuts

While growing up, Josephine and her siblings ate roasted peppernuts to become immune to flu and bad colds. As a child, she learned to fix the peppernuts herself.

Josephine usually gathers peppernuts in the middle of October, right after hunting season, when they fall from the trees. The harvest varies from year to year and tree to tree. As with acorns: *They always say every four years is a good nut crop.*

After arriving home from the harvest, Josephine squeezes the nuts out of their outer, soft hull, which she considers too bitter to eat. The skin's oily residue helps seal the shell, so the nuts keep longer. *I've had a lot of nuts here for three or four years.*

Josephine places the nuts several deep, or about one-and-a-half inches thick, in three special "*boxes*" she once used for sifting clay when she belonged to a Hoopa-based pottery guild. The boxes consist of a 12 x 12 frame of boards about six inches high with a screen that runs underneath. Josephine sun-dries the nuts during the day, propping the boxes up off the ground with sticks, so there's ample ventilation through the screen. To ensure that all the nuts dry well, she periodically stirs them and brings the boxes in at night. Once dry, after about two weeks, Josephine transfers the nuts into a cardboard box, bag or jar—whatever's available for storage. Alternatively, dry the nuts in a basket one nut-layer thick for three to four days before roasting.

Stored in the shell, the nuts stay "*soft,*" or, put another way, don't get "*too old.*" Josephine begins eating hers about a month after gathering them, nearer the cold and flu season. The nuts will keep for a year.

Roast peppernuts in a 250 degree oven in a pie tin or on a cookie sheet for forty-five minutes to an hour. Open the oven every five to ten minutes or so, and shake the cookie sheet so the nuts roll: *It takes the bitterness out if you cook it slow. We keep shaking them up so they roast evenly.* Without shaking, the nuts may burn on one side.

Josephine determines when the nuts have been properly roasted by the color of the shell, which turns from a yellowish tan to a light brownish-black to a dark brown. Although hot when first removed, the nuts cool fairly quickly. If cooked too long, they'll burn, which will ruin their flavor. Cooked properly, they retain a slight hint of their original bitterness, but nothing that detracts from the taste. Josephine cracks the thin shells with her teeth. The nut separates into two halves. A papery skin between the halves comes right off.

Peppernuts taste similar to a coffee bean. Eat the roasted nuts within a season. They absorb moisture through the shell and eventually become soft and chewy, which damages the taste. Josephine stores roasted ones in a jar. She eats hers plain, or, when she dishes up acorn soup, she garnishes it with roasted peppernut halves. While younger people aren't used to eating theirs this way, the "*old timers*" remember and relish it.

Pine Nuts

Josephine gathers pine nuts before the autumn rains, since rain water causes pitch to seep inside the cones, causing them to mildew and blacken. Josephine uses gloves when gathering the sharp, pitchy cones, which she transports in a cardboard box. Josephine eats the thin-shelled nuts of piñon pine. She saves the hard-shelled, tiny-seeded nuts of gray pine for jewelry and regalia making.

Seaweed

Seaweed is picked from the rocks during May's two low tides. But: *You've got to watch the tide. You've got to be quick out there.* Size is also important. *Avoid picking the big ones: If it gets too big, it's tough. You can't eat it. It's like eating kelp.*

Years ago, Josephine explained, people gathered seaweed into open-weave baskets, then rinsed it in sea water to remove any shell and sand: *You just take it out and wash it in the water. We've got our burden baskets with holes, and we just washed it in the ocean.*

Next, they formed the seaweed into cakes some eight to ten or twelve inches across, laying these on driftwood logs to dry in the sun: *We have to dry it to keep it from spoiling. The wind dried it. It'll shrink right down when it dries... [W]e just take it and put it in a [paper] bag, and save it.*

Today, so much garbage and so many pollutants have entered the ocean that Josephine would bring tap water to the beach from home. At most, she'd bring five gallons in a lard container. She would add about one-quarter cup of salt for every gallon of water and use this to rinse off any barnacles or other debris. Alternatively, clean creek water may be used for rinsing seaweed onsite. Obtain this water where the creek flows onto the beach, so it will be salty, from ocean water flowing upstream at high tides.

Some people would camp out at the beach for the two days necessary for the seaweed to fully dry. Josephine would lay hers out until evening, and then bring it home, where she could continue drying it. Whenever the beach did not get full sun, Josephine hauled the seaweed home unrinsed.

Josephine would bring extra wet seaweed home to give to people who could not gather it themselves. For herself, she generally would keep about six to seven cakes worth of seaweed.

Some haul their harvest home wet in metal buckets, tubs, clean garbage cans, and plastic bags. Josephine prefers to use a basket she loads into the back of a pickup truck. Once home, she often places the seaweed in an openwork basket some fifteen inches in diameter. The weave is close enough that she can use the same basket to clean huckleberries (see below), and, covering the basket with a cloth, leach acorn flour. When Josephine has only a little seaweed, and plans to eat it within a week, she runs tap water directly over the seaweed to rinse it off, taking care not to rinse it too much, so it retains its salt. When she has a lot of seaweed, and plans to keep it for awhile, she adds salt to the tap water.

Josephine commonly forms the seaweed into cakes and lays these on paper towels inside her home to dry: *It'll dry in two to three days.* Alternatively, she puts her seaweed cakes outside to dry on newspaper in the sun, bringing them in at night. Cakes are stored in glass gallon jars. About a dozen cakes can fit in a gallon jar, safe from moisture. They dry down to "*almost nothing.*"

Cook when fresh or dry, but don't soak it in water. When wet, cook as is (without forming into cakes) in a cast iron skillet, the type Josephine grew up with. Heat the pan without grease or oil: *Throw it in whole and toss it around until crispy.*

For taste, fry seaweed in bacon grease, just enough to cover the bottom of a cast iron skillet. The grease has to be very hot. Fry about one minute on each side, then remove with any kind of a spoon. After removing the fried seaweed, don't drain off the grease: *When we've got seaweed, we can eat it every day... If we've got bacon grease, we just throw it in the bacon grease quick, and just tip it around, then take it out and eat it. It's nice and crispy. It's got that bacony taste to it. You've got to do it quick. Just flip it in and turn it over. It's just really crispy. [....] You've got to eat it right away.*

OTHER FOODS

Fruit Butters

Josephine's mother made apple and peach butters. When she ran out of sugar, she made the butters without it: *A long time ago, it was hard to get sugar. You had to work from payday to payday.*

Josephine continues to make all three fruit butters. Her nieces and nephews pitch in and peel the fruit by the five-gallon bucketful. After peeling, Josephine boils the fruit with sugar and spices, generally in the cool of the evening. Since peaches and pears are already rather sweet, she adds just enough sugar to preserve the fruit. As for spices: *For the apple and peach I put cinnamon and nutmeg. For the pears I just put nutmeg. Sometimes I put a little pinch of cloves in it, but for some reason, a lot of people don't like cloves... Some are allergic to it.* Once the fruit is cooked, Josephine cans the butters.

Salsa

Peel and chop "*lots*" of tomatoes, and let them sit overnight so the water comes to the top. Skim off the water with a ladle. Blend an onion, a long-tube yellow pepper, a bell pepper, two hot peppers, a little cilantro, and three cloves of garlic to "*make it good and tasty.*" Stir this mix into the tomatoes. Let the salsa steam overnight on the back of a woodstove until it becomes thick. On a modern stove, simmer for four or five hours. Transfer into pint jars.

Tomatoes

Can tomatoes plain. If desired, add half a teaspoon of salt per quart jar. To stew, add a little onion and celery.

Pickle Lily

Josephine's mother ran green tomatoes and cucumbers through an old hand grinder, using about a quarter as much cucumber. She added a little vinegar. Pickle lily tastes especially good with beans, meat, or fish.

Chowchow

"Chowchow" may be an Indian word. Josephine's mother ran red tomatoes through an old hand grinder. She added some kind of spice. Josephine's brother called it "chile haha." *Chowchow* tastes especially good with beans, meat, or fish.

Sourdough Pancakes

Josephine's mother made sourdough in an old crock pitcher that someone gave the family.

CHAPTER FOUR

The Plants

The information in this book is primarily for reference and education. It is not intended to be a substitute for the advice of a physician. The editors do not advocate self diagnosis or self-medication; they urge anyone with continuing symptoms, however minor, to seek medical advice. The reader should be aware that any plant substance, whether used as food or medicine, externally or internally, may cause an allergic reaction in some people.

PLANT LISTINGS

On the following pages, you'll find a complete list of the plants Josephine uses, alphabetized according to the common name that she most prefers, followed by other common names that Josephine uses, when she uses more than one. In those instances where the plant is more widely known by an alternative common name, this name is included as an "aka."

Each plant listing includes information about whether the plant is native or non-native, the part or parts used, the purpose or purposes of a given plant's use, preparation guidelines, and, in the case of all medicinal uses, the adult dosage. You'll find additional information at the end of each entry about how Josephine first learned about a given plant, and stories related to the plant's growth and use. These stories are repeated in abbreviated form after every plant for which the information applies.

PLANT IDENTIFICATION

This book is not intended as a guide to plant identification. To ensure correct identification, each plant listing includes the plant's Latin binomial. In some cases, the Latin name of the particular species that Josephine uses is not known; this is indicated by the abbreviation "sp." In other cases, more than one species is used; this is indicated by the abbreviation "spp." For example, "*Arctostaphylos* spp." indicates that two or more species are used, but it is not known which species Josephine prefers.

The scientific names follow *The Jepson Manual* (Hickman 1993). As often as possible, plant specimens gathered by or with Josephine were used for determining the scientific names. In other instances, the plants were gathered by others, then brought to Josephine. Josephine confirmed a few plant identifications by examining printouts of photographs from *CalPhotos* online, www.calphotos.berkeley.edu.

Plant specimens were often collected from nearby locations rather than from Josephine's customary gathering areas. These plant specimens will be housed at the Humboldt State University Vascular Plant Herbarium in Arcata, California.

KARUK NAMES

James A. Ferrara (n.d. and 2004) compiled and edited the Karuk names listed in the text. Karuk elder Violet Super served as his primary cultural consultant. The Karuk Tribe of California holds the copyright to this material. In addition to the names they had for native plants, the Karuk had names for several non-native plants that became naturalized in their homeland.

The common names used by Ferrara in his publications have been modified for consistency with those used by Josephine. The Latin binomials have been modified for consistency with those used by *The Jepson Manual*. The English glosses, when known, have been provided in brackets. In some cases, where the Karuk name of a given plant isn't known, but that of a closely related plant is, the latter is listed, along with its common name and Latin binomial.

Where the Karuk name of a given plant, or a closely related one, isn't known, the "Karuk Name" heading is omitted.

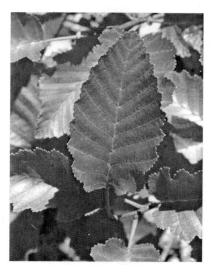

White alder. Photo by Jennifer Kalt.

Alder, white

KARUK NAME: akvíttip

LATIN NAME: *Alnus rhombifolia*

NATIVE PLANT: Yes

PART USED: Fresh, small stems usually used, although the bark may also be used.

USE: Builds the lungs and, thereby, physical strength. Good for TB.

PREPARATION: Gather the small stems or chip off the bark with a small axe. Chop into small pieces, lay out to dry, then store in jars. Steep as a tea.

DOSAGE: Make a quart of the tea and drink it, spaced out, over a day and a half. The amount of alder used doesn't make a difference. Sometimes Josephine steeps a good handful in a quart of water. She strives to make the tea strong, as the stems don't color the water very much.

Josephine uses white alder. Red alder (*Alnus rubra*) grows closer to the coast. Josephine, who used to live near the Hoopa Valley hospital, recalls the prevalence of tuberculosis, now a thing of the past: *A lot of it was cured by drinking that* [alder tea]. White alder tea was often used in conjunction with tanoak acorns: *With boys that are wrassling and running, you give them acorns to build up their strength. We use the alder bark to make a tea that strengthens their lungs... I took it for a while because my lungs were bad...a couple of years ago* [circa 1999]... *A long time ago, they used to have marathons. They ran for miles, and they always took that. They'd give them acorns, and then alder bark tea.*

The marathons of old to which Josephine refers here include the 1927 and 1928 Redwood Empire Marathon, a 462-mile, promotional run from San Francisco to Grants Pass, Oregon, designed to encourage tourism along the recently completed Redwood Highway, and featuring American Indian runners, including John Southard and Henry Thomas, both Karuk, the winners of the first and second marathons respectively. The 1928 run was the last, due to the Depression (Torliatt 2001:113-118).

See also: tanoak.

Alfalfa

LATIN NAME: *Medicago sativa*

NATIVE PLANT: No, but locally cultivated.

PART USED: The whole plant before it blossoms.

USE: This extremely nutritive plant, with its high level of chlorophyll, alkalizes, detoxifies, and clears cholesterol out of the bloodstream. It's a "fat splitter," used to break up clogged arteries. It decreases the desire for alcohol and plant-based drugs, but does not have this effect on more modern, chemically-derived drugs. Useful for the pituitary gland and arthritis. Also useful for gingivitis, which is caused by eating a lot of grapes and acidic fruits.

PREPARATION: Gather only organically-grown alfalfa that hasn't been sprayed. Pick alfalfa when it is about eight inches tall, before it blooms. Used fresh or, more commonly, dry. Drink as a tea, except for gingivitis, in which case chew fresh or dried. Saliva softens alfalfa.

DOSAGE: Use the standard dosage of one teaspoon to one cup of hot water. Drink as much as you want two to three times per day: *It won't hurt them.*

Josephine prefers fresh alfalfa: *You can buy it in a health food store in tea bags, but I'd rather get it fresh, if you can find a nice field away from the highways, where it's not sprayed.* Alfalfa tea contains seven different kinds of vitamins and minerals. A Yurok friend gathers alfalfa for Josephine from a field where it's organically grown. The tea helps Josephine sleep.

At the Old Home Place, Josephine's family raised alfalfa for their cattle and horses: *We used to like the taste of it. They always said to chew the alfalfa raw in our teeth.* Josephine's father explained to them that it keeps the teeth from rotting. He teased them with the admonition, "You never saw a cow have a heart attack."

See also: Redmond clay and hops.

Apple, domestic

LATIN NAME: *Malus* spp.

NATIVE PLANT: No, but locally cultivated.

PART USED: Sap from inner bark.

USE: Boils, bee stings, insect and spider bites. Fruit made into butters, duff and pies.

PREPARATION: For boils and insect strings, chop off a piece of the bark, collect the juice that flows from the inner bark, and apply. For food recipes, see the subsection on jams and jellies in the cooking with fruit section of "Native Plant Foods"; the subsections on duff, pie, and fried pies in the pastry section of "Native Plant Foods"; and the section on fruit butters in "Other Foods."

DOSAGE: N/A

As children, Josephine and her siblings ran barefooted through the family's alfalfa fields and inevitably got stung. The kids would gather apple juice and apply it themselves. Josephine also learned about apple from Phoebe Maddux, a Karuk midwife who showed Josephine "*a lot of things.*"

Artichoke

LATIN NAME: *Cynara scolymus*

NATIVE PLANT: No, but locally cultivated.

PART USED: Artichoke leaf and wormwood tops (stem, leaves, and flowers).

USE: Treating cow and horse flukes.

PREPARATION: If dry, soak the artichoke leaf and wormwood tops to soften. Mash into a paste, apply, then cover with a "*big band-aid.*"

DOSAGE: Leave in place overnight.

Josephine's uncle had horses, and her own family had cows, so she saw people using this remedy a long time ago. The flukes appear as a lump underneath the skin.

Artichoke, Jerusalem

aka sunroot, sunchoke, and topinambur, common names that Josephine does not use

LATIN NAME: *Helianthus tuberosus*

NATIVE PLANT: No, but native to the eastern United States.

PART USED: Tuber

USE: Diabetes

PREPARATION: Eat plain, cut up into salads, or cooked in stews and soups.

DOSAGE: Eat as much as you like.

When Josephine was growing up, there was no name for diabetes. Josephine thinks that what the locals called dropsy in the old days was actually diabetes. She recalls a relative who died of dropsy whose leg turned black and needed amputation. The use of this plant for treating diabetes is one particular to Josephine. She has not used it in some time.

Banana

LATIN NAME: *Musa* spp.

NATIVE PLANT: No

PART USED: Peel

USE: Elimination of old-age spots.

PREPARATION: Cut little squares of peel and bandage with the inside of the peel against the skin.

DOSAGE: As the peel dries, keep changing as needed until the spots are gone. Josephine learned about banana from the Native doctors in South America.

Barberry

aka tall Oregon grape, a common name that Josephine does not use

KARUK NAME: thukinpirish (*B. aquifolium*) ["bile-plant"]

LATIN NAME: Probably *Berberis aquifolium*.

NATIVE PLANT: No, but naturalized in North America.

PART USED: Upper part of plant.

USE: Laxative, typhoid, jaundice, appetite improvement, promotion of bile-secretion.

PREPARATION: Make a tea.

DOSAGE: Steep one half teaspoon to one cup of hot water. Take one half cup morning and evening. As a laxative, take a strong cupful, about one tablespoon of herb to one cup of hot water.

Josephine has experimented with barberry, which grows in Oregon, for treating her own diabetes, but has otherwise not used it: *They get the leaves and chop them up a little... [Y]ou can see stems in it... Different ones smoked it, too. I*

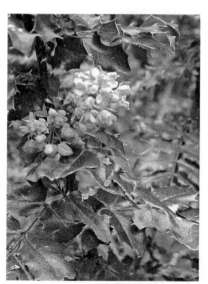
Barberry (*Berberis aquifolium var. aquifolium*). Photo by Jennifer Kalt.

don't know the reason they smoked it. It must've been tobacco... I've seen them use it around here... It comes in... It's almost like a blood purifier. It's good for a lot of things. But we don't use it too much here, because we've got our own types of herbs...

Berberis aquifolium root was identified by Karuk cultural consultants[26] as "a good medicine in all kinds of sickness," when boiled for a tea. The leaves and roots were used with other herbs to create a healing steam (Schenck and Gifford 1952:383). *Berberis vulgaris* is sold commercially as barberry.

Big-leaf maple

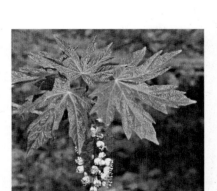

Big-leaf maple leaves and flower clusters. Photo courtesy East Bay Regional Park District Botanic Garden.

KARUK NAME: sáan ["leaf"]

LATIN NAME: *Acer macrophyllum*

NATIVE PLANT: Yes

PART USED: Leaves

USE: To keep insects out of dried eel or fish.

PREPARATION: Place fresh leaves in paper bag that has been "*closed up good.*" To dry the leaves, place the bag behind the woodstove. Put dried eel or fish in the bag with the dried leaves.

DOSAGE: N/A

As long as the eel or fish remains dry, it can keep indefinitely, although it "*gets strong after a while.*" In Jo's experience, the eel or fish stored with big-leaf maple usually doesn't last more than three or four days, because "*everybody wants to eat it.*" For long-term storage of eel or fish, dry it thoroughly, stuff pieces in a jar, close the jar, then place it in a pan of water in the oven for an hour, until it "*seals up good.*"

Blackberry, wild (California blackberry), and Himalaya berry

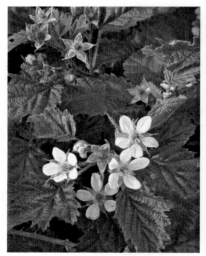

Wild blackberry. Photo by Jennifer Kalt.

KARUK NAME: attaychúrip (*R. ursinus*) ["salmon-eggs" + -chur: ? + "bush"] [-*ip*: "-bush"]

LATIN NAME: *Rubus ursinus* (wild blackberry), *Rubus discolor* (Himalaya berry)

NATIVE PLANT: Yes, and no, but naturalized and locally grown.

PART USED: Berries, young shoots.

USE: Food: Fruit eaten fresh, canned, as a jelly with wild blackberries, and as duff, pie, and fried pies. Peeled young shoots eaten fresh.

PREPARATION: Eat ripe berries. For information about gathering, cleaning, and storing the berries, see the section on fruit in "Native Plant Foods." For information about wild blackberry and Himalaya berry food preparation, see the subsections on canned fruit, and jams and jellies, in the cooking with fruit section of "Native Plant Foods"; and the subsections on duff, pie, and fried pie, in the pastry section of "Native Plant Foods." Peel the new shoots of blackberry, and eat what remains. Josephine describes the taste as "*odd*" and "*sour,*" like pond lily.

DOSAGE: N/A.

See also: lily, pond.

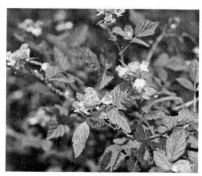

Blackcap. Photo by Beverly Ortiz.

Blackcap (wild raspberry), and domestic red raspberry

KARUK NAME: *paturúpveen'ippa(ha)* (*R. leucodermis*) ["raspberry-bush"]

LATIN NAME: *Rubus leucodermis* (blackcap), probably *Rubus idaeus* (domestic red raspberry)

NATIVE PLANT: Yes and no, respectively.

PART USED: Leaves for medicine; shoots and berries for food.

USE: Used to treat mouth sores, mouth cankers, gum boils (pyorrhea), fever blisters from eating acidic foods, and sore throats. Fresh and dried leaves and their stems used to make a gargle for sore throat. Inside of new shoots eaten. Fruit eaten fresh, and as jelly, pie, and fried pies.

PREPARATION: Gather fresh leaves for mouth sores, mouth cankers, gum boils, and fever blisters: *They grow wild in swamps and wherever it's wet along the roads.*

For a gargle, boil a quart of water, turn off the heat, and pour the water immediately onto a handful of the leaves. Add a little salt. Steep as strong a gargle as you can handle. For preparation details, see the section on gargles in "Types of Medicinals."

Peel the outer skin off the new shoots, then eat the inside. Eat ripe berries. For information about gathering, cleaning, and storing the berries, see the section on fruit in "Native Plant Foods." For information about blackcap and domestic red raspberry food preparation, see the subsection on jams and jellies in the cooking with fruit section of "Native Plant Foods"; and the subsections on pie and fried pie in the pastry section of "Native Plant Foods." Recalls Josephine: *That was really something when we could pick enough to make a pie.*

DOSAGE: Chew the fresh leaves for mouth sores, canker sores, gum boils, and fever blisters: *When you dry it, it takes too much out of it.* One cannot overdose on this plant, so, Josephine has no recommended amount to chew: *Just grab a bunch.* Chew the leaves two or three times a day, especially after meals.

Gargle about a quarter of a cup two or three times a day, with the water as hot as you can stand. Reheat as needed.

Eat fresh berries with restraint, lest they cause mouth sores.

Like ginseng, raspberry strengthens the uterine wall. Like strawberry and blackcap, it's useful for gum sores or blisters. Josephine uses whichever herb is handiest when she needs it.

When Josephine was a child, her mother treated tonsillitis with iodine dipped onto homemade swabs made of cotton on a long stick. Josephine's preferred sore throat remedy is seaweed, due to its iodine content.

Josephine ate the inside of the young shoots of blackcap as a child.

Eating grapes and cherries in the spring, as well as fresh walnuts, will also result in mouth sores.

See also: ginseng and strawberry.

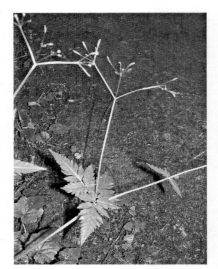

Black jack (*Osmorhiza* sp.).
Photo by Jennifer Kalt.

Black jack (California licorice, sweet cicely)

KARUK NAME: imkanva'uxpirishpirishhitihan (*O. berteroi*) ["having-leaves-like-Bitter-Greens"] múhish (*O. occidentalis*) ["its-seeds"]

LATIN NAME: *Osmorhiza berteroi* (synonym *O. chilensis*)

NATIVE PLANT: Yes

PART USED: Above-ground plant, including the seeds.

USE: Childhood drink.

PREPARATION: Put plant in water for the drink.

DOSAGE: N/A

Black jack, with its long, thin, black seeds, is similar in appearance to angelica. It shouldn't be confused with dog fennel (*Anthemis cotula*), a naturalized pasture weed with a distasteful smell. *Osmoriza occidentalis* also grows in the local area.

Josephine and her siblings used to make their black jack drink for fun: *We used to chew it, and play with it, and drink it all the time* [laughs], *because it had a good taste* [laughs].

We used to have licorice gum a long time ago. You could buy it… I remember my aunt had this store we used to buy it from. Black jack gum, like this plant, tasted like black licorice.

Blood root

LATIN NAME: *Sanguinaria canadensis*

NATIVE PLANT: No, but native to the eastern United States.

PART USED: Root

USE: Used to dissolve tumors and shrink goiters.

PREPARATION: Take as drops or in ought capsules. Add a pinch of peppermint or spearmint for taste.

DOSAGE: Put fifteen drops of liquid blood root obtained in a health food store in a teaspoon of water and take twice a day for five days. Do not exceed this dosage, as the drops are very concentrated. Stop for two or three days, then repeat. It takes five to six weeks to dissolve a tumor.

Alternatively, due to the herb's bad taste, place the pounded root in ought capsules. Take two capsules a day, one in the morning, the other in the evening. For goiter, take the same way, three times per week, until the goiter recedes.

Josephine uses blood root to shrink brain tumors, although it can shrink other tumors as well. Josephine trades for blood root from back east (Vermont and North Carolina). She learned about this plant from another Indian doctor.

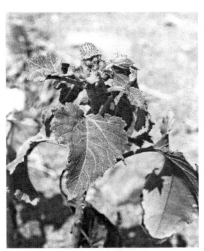

Burdock. Photo by Beverly Ortiz.

Burdock

aka cocklebur, a common name that Josephine does not use

LATIN NAME: *Xanthium strumarium*

NATIVE PLANT: Yes

PART USED: Stem before the burrs form, and the root for winter use.

USE: For purifying blood and healing burns.

PREPARATION: If the root is large, cut it in half and lay it out to dry with the centers facing up. For purifying blood, steep the stem or root in hot water until the color changes. Alternatively, put the powdered root in ought capsules.

For healing burns, powder the root in a mini-food mill, mix with boiling water, and poultice.

DOSAGE: When taking burdock for this purpose, steep a teaspoon in one cup of hot water and drink twice a day. Alternatively, take in capsules twice a day for six weeks.

For poultice, apply as with acorn flour. Wrap and leave on for two days to ease pain and prevent blistering. If the burn is deep, change the poultice twice a day for three or four days, then air the burn area and apply Vitamin E to prevent scarring.

Burdock grows along river bars and sand banks. Dogs and cats pick up the long, brown burrs in their fur.

Josephine has always been aware of burdock root as a blood purifier. Due to burdock's bitter taste, Josephine takes Oregon grape as a blood purifier instead. When Josephine was growing up, her mother used whatever blood purifier was available, mostly Oregon grape root.

See also: acorn.

Caraway, wild

LATIN NAME: Probably *Ligusticum californicum*. A pressed plant specimen labeled by Josephine as wild caraway, might be *Osmorhiza occidentalis* or *L. grayi*.

NATIVE PLANT: Yes

PART USED: Skin on carrot-like bulb; seeds when bulb unavailable.

USE: Wild caraway tea settles the stomach and enables cancer-and HIV/AIDS-patients to hold down their food.

PREPARATION: After digging the bulb, the oily-feeling skin will slip off. Steep as a tea. Alternatively, steep the seeds as a tea.

DOSAGE: Use one teaspoon per cup of water. Drink the tea about thirty minutes before eating.

Josephine has always known this plant: *Some people call the wild caraway root angelica, but it's not. It has the same type of flowers and leaves.*

Catnip

LATIN NAME: Probably *Nepeta cataria*

NATIVE PLANT: European, but locally naturalized.

PART USED: Root

USE: Used by Josephine for gas pains. Also used for convulsions in children, colic, and to induce sleep. Soothing to the nerves.

PREPARATION: Let the root dry to reduce the juice, but not so much that it becomes hard. Next, pound up the root, then store it.

DOSAGE: Steep one teaspoon of the pounded root in one cup of hot water.

Catnip grows in moist areas along roadsides. The root is smaller than that of wild ginger.

See also: ginger.

Cayenne (capsicum, hot pepper)

LATIN NAME: *Capsicum annuum*

NATIVE PLANT: No

PART USED: Pod

USE: Stimulates healing of internal bleeding ulcers, because it gets the blood flowing around the sore. Used for poor circulation, heart trouble and dropsy. Used with lobelia, a relaxant, for people experiencing a lot of pain, as from ulcers.

PREPARATION: Put in ought capsules due to bad taste.

DOSAGE: Take one capsule per day until circulation improves (you start warming up). Due to the dangerous qualities of lobelia, the dosage for those experiencing severe pain has been withheld.

Josephine acquires cayenne in strings from Taos, or in powdered form. Various people bring it to her. Lorencita "Boots" Masten (Tewa), the Hoopa school cook, used to give capsicum to Jo.

Boots was born in 1907 in the Pueblo of San Juan, New Mexico. Orphaned at age six, she attended grammar school at an Indian boarding school in Santa Fe. Upon Boots' high school graduation from an Indian boarding school in Albuquerque, she accepted a position as cook at the then Hoopa government school, a position which the Albuquerque school superintendent told her about. She arrived in Hoopa on October 8, 1928, serving as cook until her retirement in 1969 (Anonymous 1980: 8,11). Boots gave cayenne, purchased in cans, to people with poor circulation. She'd form it into a ball, then instruct them to swallow it quickly. Relatives in New Mexico also sent Josephine capsicum strings.

Before capsules were available, capsicum was added to foods during the cooking process, such as salsas.

Josephine prefers shepherd's purse for bleeding ulcers. Place the stem and heart-shaped leaf of shepherd's purse in boiling water. It will gel after it cools. Take to coat the stomach.

When Josephine was growing up, there was no name for diabetes. Josephine thinks that what the locals called dropsy in the old days was actually diabetes.

See also: lobelia and shepherd's purse.

Cheeseweed (mallow)

LATIN NAME: *Malva parviflora.*

NATIVE PLANT: No, but locally naturalized.

PART USED: Whole plant (roots, stems, leaves) with or without the flower, but especially the seed capsule (fruit) and its encircling leaves. Josephine keeps the chopped up root in a jar.

USE: For kidneys and urine leakage (where blood in the urine blocks the passage) cheeseweed acts to clean out any blockages in the passages. Used to treat lung blockages: asthma, bronchial trouble (caused by colds), emphysema, and pneumonia. Also used for blistering in the mucous membranes of the mouth, caused by eating acidy foods or too many fresh walnuts.

PREPARATION: Caution: Do not take if pregnant: *You're not supposed to take it when you're pregnant, because it'll abort.*

For all uses, steep as a tea in the standard ratio of a teaspoon to one cup of hot water: *You can make it light...just like ordinary tea. You don't get it too strong to start with.* For gargle, make stronger. For preparation details, see the section on gargles in "Types of Medicinals."

DOSAGE: For kidneys and urine blockages, drink once a day for about a week. For asthma, about a cup should be sufficient, as the attacks don't last long. For bronchial trouble, take less than a cup a day for about a week. For emphysema and pneumonia, drink a quarter of a cup at a time about three times a day. Continue while you have the condition, but for no more than three days. With emphysema, it merely relieves the symptoms. For mucous membranes, gargle two times a day for two days, the stronger the tea the better.

The name of this plant derives from the "cheesy taste" of its fruit: *I have* [cheeseweed] *growing out around the chicken yard. I see it grow out here in the front. We cut it down a lot of times... It generally grows around barns, I guess where it gets a lot of manure. Inside of the flower, there'll be a little six-sided, flat fruit that'll come after the bloom drops off. If it gets too hot, they die down before the flower drops off. It doesn't form that little fruit unless you find it in a shady spot.* As children, Josephine and her siblings enjoyed eating the fruits.

When Josephine was growing up, cheeseweed tea was used to treat tuberculosis, although Josephine has never used it for this purpose: *I used to see them make a tea and give it to people out here that had tuberculosis. We had lots of tuberculosis way back in the twenties... Mountain balm is used for tuberculosis, too...*

See also: mountain balm.

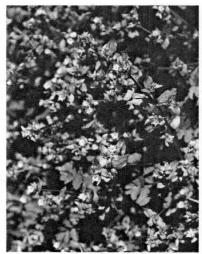

Chickweed. Photo by Beverly Ortiz.

Chickweed

LATIN NAME: *Stellaria media*

NATIVE PLANT: No, but locally naturalized.

PART USED: Use the whole plant, except the root, including the flowers.

USE: Laxative. Cleanses the system.

PREPARATION: Gather in the spring. Always use this juicy plant fresh. To cleanse the system, add to salads or sandwiches in the spring, when the plant is out.

DOSAGE: After eating as much chickweed as you can for two days, begin six weeks on a blood purifier.

Although other chickweed species grow locally, some native, some not, Josephine uses chickweed as the name for the species that grows in her yard.

Chickweed contains the same nutrients as miner's lettuce and is used the same way.

See also: miner's lettuce and psyllium.

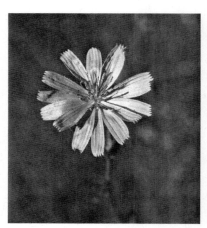

Chicory. Photo by Beverly Ortiz.

Chicory

LATIN NAME: *Cichorum intybus*

NATIVE PLANT: No, but locally naturalized.

PART USED: Root

USE: Good for people with jaundice. Works on the spleen, pancreas, liver, and kidneys.

PREPARATION: Dig the root, which is common locally. Split it open and dry it. Steep as a tea. For coffee, chop the root into small pieces and roast it in a glass or Pyrex pan in the oven at about 250 degrees for about fifteen to twenty minutes. Every two minutes or so, open up the oven and stir the chicory to prevent it from burning on one side. Place the roasted root in a pot of water on the stove. Bring water to a boil, then turn off the heat (don't steep the root).

DOSAGE: Use the standard dosage of a teaspoon to one cup, but only drink a half a cup, once a day, for about a week, then quit for two days. If still needed, resume taking.

While Josephine was always aware that this plant could be used as a tea, she drank it for the first time at a doctoring conference in Bogotá, Columbia, where chicory coffee was served: *Down there they gave us a fancy teacupful.*

The stool will look like white, shredded coconut after three days.

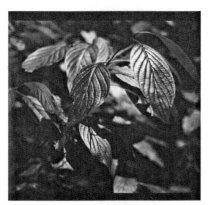

Chitem bark. Photo by Beverly Ortiz.

Chitem bark (cascara)

aka cascara buckthorn, a common name that Josephine does not use

KARUK NAME: xutyúppin

LATIN NAME: *Rhamnus purshiana*

NATIVE PLANT: Yes

PART USED: Leaves, stems, bark.

USE: Laxative and liver cleanser.

PREPARATION: Break up the leaves and stems, which can be used dry or fresh. Steep as a tea in the ratio of one teaspoon to one cup of hot water.

DOSAGE: Take judiciously; use about a shot glassful. For liver cleanser, take half a cup.

The old people called this plant "chitem bark." *It's bad tasting. Every time we got sick when we were young, we had to take that.* During World War II, the locals were paid to strip the bark off the trees and bag it up for use as a laxative. They'd travel to Eureka with the bark, where it was sold to a buyer.

Wild choke-cherry. Photo courtesy East Bay Regional Park District Botanic Garden.

Choke-cherry, wild (wild cherry)

aka western choke-cherry, a common name that Josephine does not use

KARUK NAME: púun

LATIN NAME: *Prunus virginiana* var. *demissa*

NATIVE PLANT: Yes

PART USED: Both the inner and outer bark of these thin-barked plants. The medicine resides in the sap and juice of the inner bark.

USE: Mix choke-cherry bark with mountain balm and heal-all for cough, asthma, bronchitis, whooping cough, and pneumonia syrup. Mixed with dogwood, choke-cherry is used for heart ailments. The mixture of the two barks lowers blood pressure and regulates the heartbeat: [It] *increases the force of the heart action.*

PREPARATION: Gather the bark from the side of plant that is exposed to early morning sun. Strip off three-inch pieces of the bark in the spring, when the sap is flowing, or scrape it off at other times of the year, taking care not to take too much, or ring (girdle) the plant, which will kill it. Use fresh, or dry to store. Once the herbs have dried, she stores them in jars or paper bags in a suitcase. For details on the preparation and use of syrup, see the section on cough syrups in "Types of Medicinals." For heart ailments, use choke-cherry and dogwood bark in even amounts. Steep a teaspoonful of these barks in a pint of water: *I steep it to get everything out of the bark, then I strain it and keep it.* Josephine never makes more than a quart of this medicine, which can be set aside for use whenever one feels heart pain, or the heart races. *I generally get them in the spring when the sap's up, then dry them.*

Josephine finds choke-cherry and dogwood bark in combination better than digitalis, which is dangerous to take. She also prefers these to foxglove, which has become naturalized in the valley. *I avoid it. I'm scared of that stuff, because it can build up in your system.* To improve the taste, drink the dogwood and choke-cherry tea in orange juice.

DOSAGE: *When my heart's acting up, maybe I'll drink half a cup a day. You take it in small amounts.* You can also put the bark into ought capsules. Take one capsule with water whenever needed, but for no more than two days.

When Josephine was growing up, dogwood with choke-cherry bark was commonly used by those who had heart trouble, something that occurred on both sides of Josephine's family.

Josephine ate choke-cherry berries raw as a child, although they were somewhat bitter. *You don't find much wild cherry around any more. I have one growing in my mother's yard* [in the Hoopa Valley], *and I keep a good watch on it so nobody will cut it down or do anything with it* [laughs].

According to Schenck and Gifford (1952), in 1939, the Karuk ate the berries when ripe rather than preserving them.

See also: dogwood.

Clover, pink

KARUK NAME: axmúhishanach ichxúunanach (red clover, *T. pratense*) ["little-blood-seeded-one", "little-hatted-one"]

LATIN NAME: *Trifolium pratense*

NATIVE PLANT: No

PART USED: Flowers, above-ground plant (leaves, stems and flowers).

USE: Blood purifier

PREPARATION: Prepare fresh or dried as tea for purifying the blood.

DOSAGE: Steep one tablespoon to one cup. Strain out the plant material. There's no concern with dosage, as this plant isn't dangerous. It's scarce, however, so Josephine doesn't have much experience with it.

Pink clover has flower clusters nearly an inch across. The blossoms are a pretty pink color. Pink clover used to be common at the Old Home Place, but has been virtually eliminated from the Hoopa area, probably due to grazing.

Twenty-six clover species grow in the Klamath Ranges Floristic Province. Eight of these are non-native (*T. arvense, T. campestre, T. glomeratum, T. hybridum, T. pretense*), all native to Europe; *T. incarnatum*, native to southern Europe; *T. hirtum*, native to Eurasia and North Africa; and *T. repens*, native to Eurasia (*The Jepson Manual* on-line). Although naturalized in California, *T. pratense*, with its red-purple corolla, was apparently notable enough to achieve a Karuk name. *T. hirtum*, or rose clover, another non-native, has a generally pink corolla of the same size.

See also: alfalfa.

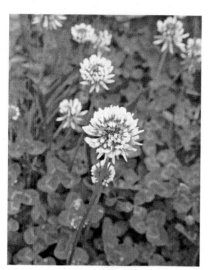

White clover. Photo by Jennifer Kalt.

Clover, white

LATIN NAME: Likely *Trifolium repens*

NATIVE PLANT: Unknown

PART USED: All of the above-ground plant (leaves, stems and flowers).

USE: Boils, ulcerated sores that don't heal, and other skin diseases. Also used for treating internal cancers and canker sores.

PREPARATION: For boils, ulcerated sores that don't heal, and other skin diseases, mash the fresh tops and apply as a poultice or, alternatively, make into a salve with plantain and dandelion. For preparation and use details, see the sections on poultices and salves in "Types of Medicinals."

For internal cancers, make tea using two or three flower tops per cup of water. A larger batch of the strained tea may be kept for a day or two. For canker sores use the whole plant to prepare a mouthwash.

DOSAGE: Apply salve periodically until sore or boil is healed. For internal cancers, take tea three times per day. Use for several weeks, or as long as needed.

For canker sores, use as a mouthwash for two or three days.

This clover, which grows in Josephine's yard, has white blossoms with pink tips. It has not been definitively keyed.

When Josephine was a child, a commercial clover salve was available: *You can buy clover in a salve... That clover salve came out years ago... You can still buy it some places... I remember a long time ago, it came in a little round flat can... We used to buy it from...the Raleigh man[27] or whoever came through. He always had it. He had a lot of liniments and Lady Pinkums. Lady Pinkums were taken by girls who started their menstrual periods that had a hard time..., and Golden Metal Discovery. Golden Metal Discovery...had all kinds of herbs [listed] on the bottle. I had nosebleeds so bad my dad used to buy it for me. It built up your blood... And he had another one, too, but I can't remember what that one was. I used to have to take it...because I'd bleed... They tried more than one thing to cure that... I was born with a blood disease... If you get bumped, you get big bruises under your skin. Even if you just barely touch it. My shins were always black and blue... I'd bleed under the skin for a long time.*

T. repens, with it's 7-11 mm. white corolla, is native to Europe, but common in the local area. *T. eriocephalum*, a common, native clover, has a dull-white to yellowish corolla, 8-14 mm. across. *T. cyanthiferum*, another native clover, has white or yellowish, pink-tipped flowers (*The Jepson Manual* on-line).

See also: plantain, ribbed and dandelion.

Cohosh, black

LATIN NAME: Unknown

NATIVE PLANT: No

PART USED: Unknown

USE: Contains female estrogen: *People going through the change of life used to take a lot of it.* Good for menopause, menstrual cramps, high blood pressure, nerves, equalizing the circulation, and relief of childbirth pain.

PREPARATION: Due to bad taste, put in double ought capsules.

DOSAGE: Take two double ought capsules a day, one in the morning, the other in the evening, for only a few days. Usually, Josephine prescribes black cohosh capsules to women in labor to relieve the pain and bleeding. For standard labor, take one; for a long labor, two.

Black cohosh used to grow in the local area, but was destroyed when an old highway was replaced. Josephine obtains hers from herbal gardeners. It appears to be a different plant from that sold as black cohosh in health food stores.

Cohosh, blue

LATIN NAME: Unknown. *Caulophyllum thalictroides*, from eastern North America, is sold commercially as blue cohosh, but is not used for the purposes for which Jo prescribes it.

NATIVE PLANT: No

PART USED: Root

USE: For high blood pressure, dropsy, diabetes, and epilepsy.

PREPARATION: Root steeped.

DOSAGE: Dosage withheld due to the dangerous qualities of this plant.

Josephine's blue cohosh gathering site was destroyed by spraying along the highways for fire prevention.

When Josephine was growing up, there was no name for diabetes. Josephine thinks that what the locals called dropsy in the old days was actually diabetes.

Coltsfoot

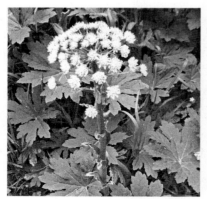

Coltsfoot. Photo by Jennifer Kalt.

LATIN NAME: *Petasites frigidus* var. *palmatus*

NATIVE PLANT: Yes

PART USED: Root

USE: Soak for swelling from star thistle "*poisoning.*" Poultice and salve for sores that don't heal (external cancerous sores, ulcerated sores, and bedsores). Salve for boils, ulcerated sores, and skin diseases.

PREPARATION: For soak, boil water, then immediately pour over coltsfoot root, and, while the water is warm, soak the swelled limb (leg, arm or hand). For preparation details, see the section on soaks in "Types of Medicinals." Although you can use the dry root, it's a little easier to use fresh.

For poultice, mash the root with a hammer, then apply.

For salve for sores that don't heal, use the root with heal-all, Johnny jump-up, and dried wormwood blossoms. For preparation details, see the section on salves in "Types of Medicinals." For salve for treating boils, ulcerated sores and skin diseases (psoriasis, scabies, mange, and ringworm), use the root with plantain (wide-leaf or ribbed), wormwood, and garden violet if pain. For preparation details, see the section on salves in "Types of Medicinals."

DOSAGE: Use until healed.

Josephine has always known about coltsfoot. This plant, which grows in damp places, has interconnected "roots" (rhizomes) from which new plants grow: *You go along maybe a foot and another growth will come out. It'll grow along, if you pull it out, maybe six or seven feet.*

See also: heal-all, Johnny-jump-up, plantain, ribbed, and wormwood.

Corn

LATIN NAME: *Zea mays*

NATIVE PLANT: No, but cultivated locally

PART USED: The tassel (silk)

USE: For kidney and bladder, prostate, painful urination. Causes bed-wetting to cease.

PREPARATION: Pull off the silk. Break up with a cleaver, or, nowadays, a chopper. Steep fresh or dried as a tea. The tea gets cloudy if stored, so make a pint at most.

DOSAGE: Use the standard dosage of one teaspoon to one cup of hot water. Take the tea twice a day for three days. For prostate concerns, take for a month.

Josephine has always known about corn silk.

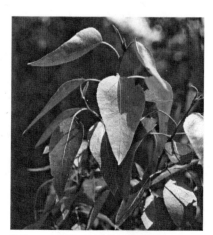
Cottonwood. Photo by Beverly Ortiz.

Cottonwood

aka black cottonwood, a common name that Josephine does not use

KARUK NAME: *asáppiip* [asa-, "rock," + -pi- (?) + -ip, "tree"]

LATIN NAME: *Populus balsamifera* subsp. *trichocarpa*

NATIVE PLANT: Yes

PART USED: "*Three brown things on tips*" of branches when they come out in the spring (February or March).

USE: Salve with mullein and ribbed plantain for sores that don't heal. Gargle for sore throat remedy with slippery elm.

PREPARATION: Pick these three pitchy parts. Save dried in a jar. For preparation details of salve, see the section on salves in "Types of Medicinals." For gargle, combine a pinch of cottonwood and slippery elm in a half cup of hot water. For preparation details, see the section on gargles in "Types of Medicinals."

DOSAGE: Use salve periodically until sores have healed.

Useful in salves and gargles due to its turpentine content.

See also: mullein, plantain, ribbed, and slippery elm.

Cranesbill (germander)

aka storksbill and filaree, common names that Josephine does not use

LATIN NAME: *Erodium botrys, brachycarpum, cicutarium,* or *moschatum.* These four species, all naturalized in northwest California, look very similar, and it is unlikely the Josephine and her siblings distinguished between them.

NATIVE PLANT: Yes

PART USED: Leaves

USE: Although Josephine hasn't used the plant medicinally, she has heard it was good for strep throat.

PREPARATION: Unknown

DOSAGE: Unknown

It has a leaf like a geranium… Sometimes we call it cranesbill.

As children, Josephine and her siblings turned the elongated fruits (capsules) into scissors, and pretended to "*scissors*" each other. Also for fun, they'd shoot the capsules at each other. When dry, they held the seed pods between their fingers and aimed them at each other's hair, taking care to avoid the eyes. The barbed pods would stick, and the hair would wrap around it: *We had nothing to play with. We had to make things to do.*

Cucumber

LATIN NAME: *Cucumis sativus*

NATIVE PLANT: No

PART USED: Fruit

USE: Sore eyes, pink eye (sties).

PREPARATION: For medicinal purposes, it's best to use the fresh, new cucumbers, rather than the old, yellow ones. Slice the fruit about an eighth of an inch thick, leaving the peel in place. Bind with gauze.

DOSAGE: For pink eye, apply twice a day, or leave on overnight.

Josephine's parents always used it for sties or pink eye. *We used to mash a whole cucumber and make a mask for the whole face.* For this purpose, peel and remove the seeds. Mash the pulp around the seeds.

As a teenager and young woman, Josephine had lots of freckles, and decided to try cucumber to remove them. Since this required a lot of cucumbers, she was cautioned: *If you're going to do that, use the old ones.* Josephine applied a cucumber mask about once a week, letting it dry as she slept, a towel beneath her head. It worked successfully.

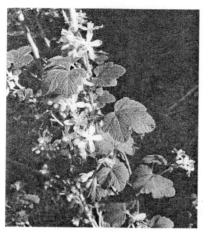

Red flowering currant.
Photo by Sydney Carothers.

Currant, red-flowering, and domestic

KARUK NAME: thuf'áhan ["mouth-of-the-creek-one"]

LATIN NAME: *Ribes sanguineum* var. *sanguineum* (red flowering currant)
Probably *Ribes nigrum* (domestic currant)

NATIVE PLANT: Yes and no, respectively.

PART USED: Fruit

USE: Used for food, not medicinally.

PREPARATION: Made into jams and jellies.

DOSAGE: N/A

Josephine's maternal grandmother and other women her age commonly planted domestic currants in their yards near the water tank, so they must have needed a lot of water to grow. They used the currants for pie, although Josephine never has.

Dahlia

LATIN NAME: *Dahlia* spp. Any species will work.

NATIVE PLANT: No, but cultivated locally.

PART USED: Bulb

USE: Diabetes

PREPARATION: Slice off a portion of the bulb

DOSAGE: *I always slice off just so much, but I never recommend it to too many people, unless they're here and see how much I take… You've got to know how much thickness to take.*

The use of this plant for diabetes is one particular to Josephine.

When Josephine was growing up, there was no name for diabetes. Josephine thinks that what the locals called dropsy in the old days was actually diabetes.

See also: Jerusalem artichoke, which is a safe alternative.

Damiana

LATIN NAME: Unknown. *Tumera diffusa* and *T. diffusa* var. *aphrodisiaca* are sold commercially as damiana.

NATIVE PLANT: No

PART USED: Top of plant (stem, leaves, flower).

USE: For sexual impotence, reproductive organs, loss of sensation and energy to limbs.

PREPARATION: Dry the plant. Steep as a tea. To smoke, crush the leaves, which have a lemony smell.

DOSAGE: Use half a teaspoon of damiana to half a cup of hot water. Start with a shot-glassful to test whether the patient's system can handle it. Increase to half a cup per day until the condition clears up. Damiana can be addictive if you take too much.

Josephine learned about this medicinal plant from Cahuilla elder Katherine Saubel: *I brought seeds up from southern California. I'm sorry I did. It's all over* [laughs]… *It's got a lemony taste… You can smoke it. I pulled one up, and it was this great, big thing… It just covered the ground. I liked the smell of it… I told my nephews, "They smoke this stuff." They tried it just one time to see what it would do* [laughs].

Dandelion

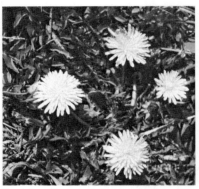

Dandelion. Photo by Deborah E. McConnell.

LATIN NAME: *Taraxacum officinale*

NATIVE PLANT: No, but locally naturalized.

PART USED: Liquid from the stems for warts. Root and leaves for water pill effects and iron anemia. Root, stem and leaves in summertime, and root in wintertime for salve.

USE: As a diuretic, for kidney and bladder problems, like taking a water pill. For treating iron anemia. For eliminating warts. For treating skin diseases (sunburn, eczema, poison oak, and psoriasis), and dry skin, such as on the elbows, make a salve with plantain and mullein. For treating skin sores (impetigo, infected sores, and ulcerated sores), make a salve with the same plants. For treating boils, sores that don't heal, and skin diseases, make a salve with plantain and white clover.

PREPARATION: Steep as a tea for water pill effects and anemia. For warts, use the fresh juice from the stems; never store the juice. Alternatively, for warts, make a salve solely with dandelion, olive oil and beeswax. For details on the preparation of salves with dandelion for treating skin diseases and skin sores, see the same section on salves.

DOSAGE: For tea, steep a teaspoon to one cup of hot water. As a diuretic, take for three days, one cup a day. For kidney and bladder complaints take for three days, twice a day. For iron anemia, take for one week. Apply salve or liquid periodically until sores or skin conditions are healed.

Sourgrass also has a water pill affect.

What's meant by kidney and bladder conditions varies. Before you can treat kidney and bladder problems, you generally have to treat the liver. *It's generally a problem in your liver that causes kidney infection.* Kidney infections primarily result from liver problems, but can sometimes be diabetes-related. Dandelion and huckleberry teas are good for treating conditions that result from diabetes. Mullein is good for bladder infection, which causes soreness.

Josephine once tried the juice on a skin spot, caused by sun exposure, and it worked.

When Josephine was growing up, to treat impetigo, she and other locals made a wash with dandelion, including the roots. They washed the dandelion and let it steep for an hour or two in hot water, strained it, then rubbed the liquid over the impetigo sores. After a day, or a day-and-a-half, they'd reapply the liquid *"just to make sure"* the sores would heal: *A long time ago in school everybody got impetigo. Of course, that's contagious.*

Although Josephine no longer remembers the details, she recalls, as a young child, making salves with her paternal grandmother.

See also: clover, white, huckleberries, mullein, turkey, plantain, ribbed, and sour-grass. For more about poison oak remedies, see also: manzanita, mullein, plantain, ribbed and wide-leaf, soaproot, Solomon seal, walnut, black, wormwood (mugwort), and oatmeal and ocean water in the non-herbal cures section.

Devil's club

LATIN NAME: *Oplopanax horridus*

NATIVE PLANT: Yes, but not locally. Grows north of Orick into British Columbia and Alaska.

PART USED: Root

USE: Blood purifier. Flu remedy. Poultices for sores and sprains: *It's going to take away that soreness, so it's got something in it for that.*

PREPARATION: Wear gloves to prevent contact with a thorny fuzz that, as Josephine describes it, "*will just eat you*": *You pull it up, and you can get one root that grows six or seven feet. One root will do you for a long time. But the natives up in Alaska cut it up and dry it.* Each root is about an inch to an inch and a quarter in diameter. Powder the root for teas. For poultices, after devil's club has been dried, put it in hot water to soak and soften: *We just use the water off of it. Soak the cloth in the water and poultice that on.* For preparation and use details, see the section on poultices in "Types of Medicinals."

DOSAGE: Take one half cup of the tea morning and evening. For blood purifier, steep one quarter teaspoon of powdered root in one half cup of boiled water for seven days, then one teaspoon in one half cup of boiled water for seven weeks, and finally four teaspoons in one half cup of boiled water for ten weeks. For flu, steep one quarter teaspoon of powdered root in one half cup of boiled water and drink the tea for ten days.

Josephine gets her devil's club, which grows in damp places, from Oregon. This plant has a hairy stem and wide leaves that resemble a hand.

Oplopanax horridus receives its name from the horrible spines that cover this plant, including its gigantic leaves. In British Columbia and Alaska devil's club is a popular medicinal: *Going up the coast into Alaska and British Columbia, it's all devil's club... It grows from Orick north. It has a big leaf on it like a thimble-berry,[28] and then in the fall, it'll have a bunch of red berries on top... One time Fred brought me some just slabbed off. He...didn't send word how to take it. I just chopped it up and made a big cupful and drank it. I went out to the chicken house and it was like I was drunk* [laughs]. *So I watched it after that. I've still got some put away somewhere* [laughs]. *They use it for everything. It's their big medicine up there... This old fellow up in Alaska, he sent it down with Fred to give to me... I used to give it down here, but...not much. Only on poulticing.*

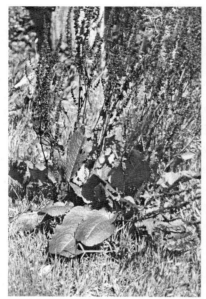

Curly dock. Photo by Beverly Ortiz.

Dock, curly (yellow dock, puke root)

KARUK NAME: chantiripirishpírishhitihan ["one-who-is-tick-leaved"]

LATIN NAME: *Rumex crispus*

NATIVE PLANT: No, but locally naturalized.

PART USED: Root.

USE: Blood purifier. Also good for tumors on glands, swelling from cancer nodes, and running sores that don't heal.

PREPARATION: Dig root in autumn after the flowers become dry. Pound the root and steep as a tea for blood purifier; poultice it for the other uses. Make the tea fresh each time. Don't store in larger batch in the refrigerator.

DOSAGE: Take moderate amounts, lest the patient vomit it up. As a blood purifier, take half a cup twice a day for four to five days, then quit for a few days, and resume taking. Take for six weeks.

Josephine had a relative who called this plant "puke root." He drank one or two cups for a hangover.

   This plant is more readily available than Oregon grape. *Any herb that turns yellow when you make a tea is good for the liver. It cleanses the liver. Like the Oregon grape root. We take that for a blood purifier. And the dock will turn pale yellow when you fix the root part.*

See also: goldenseal and Oregon grape root.

Dogwood

KARUK NAME: uyáhaama

LATIN NAME: *Cornus nuttallii*

NATIVE PLANT: Yes

PART USED: Both the inner and outer bark of these thin-barked plants.

USE: Used with choke-cherry for heart ailments caused by high blood pressure.

PREPARATION: Scrape the bark off, taking care not to ring (girdle) the plant. Use fresh, or dry to store. Use choke-cherry and dogwood bark in even amounts. Steep a teaspoonful of these barks in a pint of water: *I steep it to get everything out of the bark, then I strain it and keep it.* Josephine never makes more than a quart of this medicine, which can be set aside for use whenever one feels heart pain, or the heart races: *I generally get them in the spring when the sap's up, then dry them.* Josephine dries dogwood and other medicines by hanging them upside down on the back porch. Once the bark has dried, she stores them in jars or paper bags in a suitcase.

   Josephine finds choke-cherry and dogwood bark, in combination, better than digitalis, which is dangerous to take. She also prefers these to foxglove, which has become naturalized in the valley. *I avoid it. I'm scared of that stuff, because it can build up in your system.* For taste, drink the dogwood and choke-cherry tea in orange juice.

DOSAGE: *When my heart's acting up, maybe I'll drink a half a cup a day. You take it in small amounts. I just can't say what amounts.*

Dogwood. Photo by Jennifer Kalt.

When Josephine was growing up, dogwood and choke-cherry bark was commonly used by those who had heart trouble, something that occurred on both sides of Josephine's family.

See also: choke-cherry.

Dong quai

LATIN NAME: Unknown. *Angelica sinensis* is sold commercially as dong quai.

NATIVE PLANT: No

PART USED: Upper part of the plant. It probably doesn't make a difference if it has blooms, although Josephine acquires dong quai from others, so is unsure.

USE: This "queen of the female herbs," is used for all "female problems," including hot flashes and morning sickness. It helps to alleviate nausea from radiation therapy. It settles the stomach of HIV/AIDS patients.

PREPARATION: Use as a tea. Use the standard teaspoon to one cup of water.

DOSAGE: Drink a quarter of a cup to test for an allergic reaction in the patient. If the patient is not allergic, continue taking a quarter of a cup once daily in the morning as needed. Give to HIV/AIDS patients a half hour before they eat.

As with wild peach leaves, dong quai settles the stomach, so a patient can hold down their food.

Josephine believes she acquired knowledge of this plant's potential to alleviate nausea from radiation therapy when someone gave it to her when she was treated for a growth on her neck. *This might be something I got from the brothers.*

Echinacea

LATIN NAME: *Echinacea purpurea*. *Echinacea angustifolia, E. purpurea,* and *E. pallida* are sold commercially as Echinacea.

NATIVE PLANT: No, but locally naturalized.

PART USED: Flowers

USE: Blood purifier

PREPARATOIN: Steep as a tea.

DOSAGE: Take one teaspoon to one cup of hot water two times per day for six weeks.

Echinacea looks like a purple Shasta daisy. It grows wild in Nevada, but can now also be obtained locally. A man who runs a Weitchpec nursery brought the plants in.

Echinacea is high on Josephine's list of preferred blood purifiers. Its importance increased for her once it began to grow locally, and she learned to recognize its flowers, and so could pick it herself.

Today Josephine obtains Echinacea in powdered form.

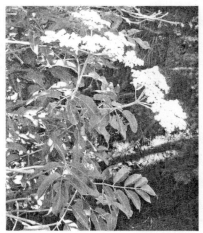

Blue elderberry. Photo by Sydney Carothers.

Elderberry, blue

LATIN NAME: *Sambucus mexicana*

NATIVE PLANT: Yes

PART USED: Inflorescence head once the little white flowers begin to fall off.

USE: Medicinal: Reduces fevers. Food: Berries eaten cooked.

PREPARATION: Steep as a tea. Elderberry tea can break a fever in a short while. Give only to adult patients, eighteen-plus years old. Give teenagers Johnny-jump-up (violet).

DOSAGE: Steep one half cup of elderberry flowers in a quart of hot water, akin to the standard teaspoon to one cup of hot water. Take one half cup. Repeat every three hours until the fever breaks. For flu, two half cups is generally enough. For smallpox and measles, healing takes longer, perhaps two to three days.

Elderberry and Johnny-jump-up work equally well for reducing fevers.

See also: Johnny-jump-up.

Eucalyptus

LATIN NAME: *Eucalyptus* spp.

NATIVE PLANT: No, but locally naturalized.

PART USED: Leaves

USE: Treating lice. Treating fleas on dogs and cats.

PREPARATION: Prepare as a rinse. For preparation and use details, see the section on rinses for hair in "Types of Medicinals."

DOSAGE: For lice, make the rinse as strong as with wormwood: *You want a dark water. We use it, then three days later, we use it again. Usually two applications will do it.* For fleas on dogs and cats, steep the leaves. Transfer enough hot water (with the leaves still in it) from the stove to fill a bucket, or to half-fill a tub, then bathe the animal in the water. Alternatively, drill the pods, string, and put them around the neck of a dog or cat.

Josephine has always known about eucalyptus, which was often put into the bed of a young animal to repel fleas. She prefers wormwood for treating lice, and reserves eucalyptus for treating fleas.

Lice and fleas were once referred to as "varmints."

Eyebright

LATIN NAME: Unknown. *Euphrasia offinale*, from Europe, sold locally as eyebright. *E. rostkoviana* is a more recent designation of the same.

NATIVE PLANT: No

PART USED: Whole, above-ground plant. It's okay to use the blossoms. Let it grow back from the roots.

USE: Clears up cataracts. Provides nutrition for the eyes, aiding sight.

PREPARATION: Use externally. Steep as a tea and use as an eyewash.

DOSAGE: Steep about one tablespoon in a pint of hot water. Rinse eyes two times a day. Continue until the condition clears up.

Josephine learned about eyebright at a doctoring conference. She used to see others using it, but didn't know why: *I knew tannin would cut cataracts.* Eyebright used to grow locally, but Josephine no longer sees it in her former gathering locales.

Fenugreek

LATIN NAME: Unknown. *Trigonella foenum-graecum* is sold commercially as fenugreek.

NATIVE PLANT: No

PART USED: Top of the plant before it flowers.

USE: Used for migraines.

PREPARATION: Prepare as tea.

DOSAGE: Use the standard dosage of a teaspoon to one cup. Start with a quarter of a cup. If it doesn't kill it, take half a cup, then quit for a while and see what it's going to do.

Josephine learned about this plant at a doctoring conference in Banff, Canada.

According to one of Josephine's many plant books, this one a plant dictionary, fenugreek is native to Southeast Europe and Western Asia. Josephine speculates: *That had to be brought over here when the Chinese came. Grindelia came over with them, the opium poppy came all the way over from the Chinese... They did a lot of mining up and down the rivers...*

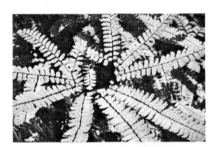
Five finger fern. Photo by Beverly Ortiz.

Fern, black (five-finger fern)

KARUK NAME: ikrittápkir yumareekrittápkir[29] ["dead-man-five-finger-fern"]

LATIN NAME: *Adiantum aleuticum*

NATIVE PLANT: Yes

PART USED: Dried or fresh leaves before the spores form.

USE: Hair rinse

PREPARATION: Steep as a tea. Use rinse after shampooing: *We just grab the top, throw it into heated up water, and steep. We always use a quart of water for a hair rinse.* For preparation details, see the section on rinses for hair in "Types of Medicinals."

DOSAGE: N/A

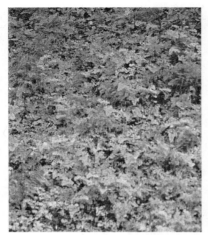

Maidenhair fern. Photo courtesy East Bay Regional Park District Botanic Garden.

Fern, maidenhair

KARUK NAME: ikrittápkir yumareekrittápkir ["dead-man-five-finger-fern"]

LATIN NAME: *Adiantum jordanii*

NATIVE PLANT: Yes

PART USED: Dried or fresh leaves before the spores form.

USE: Treating the fever of colds and flu. Also a hair rinse and conditioner: *It makes your hair really nice and soft.*

PREPARATION: Steep fresh or dried leaves as tea for colds and flu. For hair rinse, also steep as a tea. Use rinse after shampooing. *We just grab the top, throw it into heated up water, and steep. We always use a quart of water for a hair rinse.* For preparation details, see the section on rinses for hair in "Types of Medicinals."

DOSAGE: For fevers, use the standard teaspoon to one cup of hot water at least two times a day. Take three times a day if you can handle it. Take until the fever is gone. Note that some people may be allergic to this tea.

Josephine has always been aware of maidenhair fern's uses.

Fig

LATIN NAME: *Ficus carica*

NATIVE PLANT: No, but cultivated locally, and sometimes persists on its own once planted.

PART USED: Fruit, white juice for warts.

USE: Constipation, boils, carbuncles, external sores, warts, moles. When treating moles, the goal is to prevent them from becoming cancerous, although figs may also be used on moles that become neucrotic.

PREPARATION: For constipation, eat whole figs. For boils, carbuncles (a small form of boils), and other external sores, apply the white juice that's released when a fig is picked, as well as the peel of the fruit. For warts and moles, apply this same juice, which will emerge from the stem where it attaches to the fruit, as well as the broken leaves.

DOSAGE: For warts, apply the juice regularly for four or five days: *They'll just disappear all of the sudden. You don't know what happened to them... There'll be just a lot of little things coming off that make a wart. If you can get that center piece out, the wart'll just die immediately. And if you close it in and keep it from getting air, it'll die.*

Josephine's mother planted a fig at her home for medicinal purposes: *We had a lot of figs growing up... My aunt had figs down at her place, and we ate figs at the old Somes' place. When we were kids, we had lots of warts all over our fingers from playing in the old ponds* [laughs]... *We had ponds around where they placer mined...*

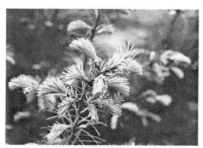

Douglas fir. Photo by Beverly Ortiz

Fir, Douglas

KARUK NAME: ithâriip ["bark-of-Douglas-fir-tree"]

LATIN NAME: *Pseudotsuga menziesii*

NATIVE PLANT: Yes

PART USED: New growth (lighter green) on tips of branches, and pitch.

USE: For tonsillitis and sore throat.

PREPARATION: Dry the new growth. Prepare a gargle. Get the water "*good and hot*" and steep. For a pint, use about ten fresh or dried fir tips (new growth). Alternatively, add pitch, taking care not to swallow when gargling. The pitch of any fir will work. Josephine lets the tea for the gargle steep for about fifteen to twenty minutes, then strains off the sticky substances through an old flour sack. For preparation details, see the section on gargles in "Types of Medicinals."

DOSAGE: You can gargle as often as you want.

A long time ago, Josephine was advised to chew pitch like a gum for sore throat, its effectiveness due to its turpentine content.

Josephine's "old granddad" said that pitch draws the electricity of lightning to it, causing the lightning to hit an "old, dry fir" in the middle: "*Well, the lightning hit an old snag, and it's burned,*" they'd say.

The small branchlets are also used as warp for fine baskets.

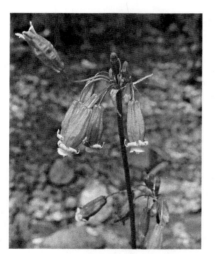

Firecracker flower. Photo courtesy East Bay Regional Park District Botanic Garden.

Firecracker flower

LATIN NAME: *Dichelostemma ida-maia*

NATIVE PLANT: Yes

PART USED: None

USE: Decoration

PREPARATION: Dig and replant.

DOSAGE: N/A

They have about an inch-long, tube flower, from one to three per plant, and they grow from a little bulb on the bottom. They used to dig it up, and plant it, to have it around the house.

Garlic

LATIN NAME: *Allium sativum*

NATIVE PLANT: No

PART USED: Fresh cloves or commercial, powdered form.

USE: Used primarily to cure hookworm infection and to control cholesterol. Emulsifies cholesterol and loosens it from arterial walls. Effective in arresting intestinal putrefaction (caused by gas), and internal infections, as from ulcers.

PREPARATION: Eat fresh for medicinal purposes. Use powdered form when cooking to flavor foods.

DOSAGE: For hookworm infection, eat one clove every day for three or four days. For other uses, also eat fresh. *It isn't going to hurt you no matter how much you take.*

Josephine has fond childhood memories of garlic, which was grown for cooking purposes in the family garden. Although it gave the children gas, they, undeterred, ate it between meals: *We always used garlic. We used to go down to the garden, pull up a bulb, and sit by the ditch and see who could eat the most garlic. We'd just bite it in two and swallow it whole. We had a race. My mom used to smell us when we got* [laughing] *back up to the house.* The family also fed their dogs fresh garlic, rolled into meat, to expel worms.

Josephine began to use garlic medicinally later in life, inspired by knowledge acquired at gatherings of Indian doctors. Josephine recalls one man who brought along big elephant garlic to one gathering. He cooked breakfast in the morning, a breakfast comprised of potatoes mixed with large amounts of cooked garlic and eggs laden with more cooked garlic: *That was quite the breakfast we had to eat* [laughs].

Elephant garlic is probably a cultivar of *A. sativum*.

Geranium (commercial)

Here Josephine refers to those species that the "*old timers*" would recognize, not the crossbred "*tame ones*" of today: *Now you don't know what* [the plant breeders are] *doing.*

LATIN NAME: *Pelargonium* spp.

NATIVE PLANT: No

PART USED: With small, garden geraniums, harvest the top of the plant, except the flowers. If the geranium is large, pluck off and use the leaves and their stems.

USE: Used for diarrhea, step throat, tonsillitis, mouth fungus, stabilizing low and high blood pressure, and virus prevention. Josephine also says: *I think geranium builds up your immune system to keep you from getting viruses...*

PREPARATION: Prepare as a tea with the standard teaspoon to one cup of hot water. For strep throat and tonsillitis, gargle with a strong tea. For preparation and use details, see the section on gargles in "Types of Medicinals." For mouth fungus, rinse mouth with the tea.

DOSAGE: For diarrhea, take two to three times a day. For blood pressure, drinking half a cup daily for five days should be adequate. For virus prevention, use several drops of the commercially available, concentrated liquid form, which Josephine purchases in health food stores. Put fifteen drops in a glass of juice. Take twice a day the first day, and one dose the second. For mouth fungus, rinse mouth two to three times a day. Don't gargle.

There's one tame geranium you can buy. If you touch the leaves, it has a really minty smell. You can use that one, too. I've forgotten what we used to call it, but Mom used to have it, and Grandma [Bennett] *used to have it... It used to bloom like a geranium, but the leaves had a nice scent. You can make tea out of it... It's just something we always had around.* Josephine has seen this cultivated variety, common in the '20s and '30s, in nurseries in Medford, Oregon.

Josephine prefers local native mushrooms for high blood pressure. Labrador tea is used for high blood pressure on the coast.

Ginger, white (wild ginger, white-veined wild ginger), and commercial ginger

White ginger. Photo by Beverly Ortiz.

LATIN NAME: *Asarum hartwegii* (white ginger)
Zingiber officinalis (commercial ginger)

NATIVE PLANT: Yes and no, respectively

PART USED: "*Root*" (rhizome)

USE: Stimulates circulation in the pelvic area. Primarily used to ease menstrual cramps. Also used for morning sickness and gas (indigestion).

PREPARATION: Wash the root, but don't remove the skin. Let it dry to reduce the sap (juice), but not so much that it becomes hard. Next, pound the root with a hammer and store it. Also use a food chopper for the latter purpose.

DOSAGE: Put a teaspoon of the pounded or chopped root in a coffee cup, then pour hot water over the top and let the mixture steep. Although strong, this is Josephine's preferred ratio of ginger to water. Drink a half cup two or three times a day. For morning sickness, add a mint leaf for taste. To alleviate gas, take one cup of white ginger tea. Add a little mint for taste. *I always put maybe three leaves in it. When you have indigestion, if you take a little bit, ginger will help with gas. We used to have a lot of peppermint, too, and that's good. Peppermint. Spearmint. Catnip. Lemon mint. Any kind will dispel the gas. Make you burp.*

A long time ago, we'd get the wild ginger, and we'd use that... If you pull it up, a root [rhizome] *will grow and start another plant. They all connect.* [....]

After moving to town, store-bought ginger (*Zingiber officinalis*) provided Josephine with an effective and available substitute for the native plant: *We'd put it in pumpkin pies.*

See also: peppermint, spearmint, catnip, and lemon mint.

Ginseng, California (elk clover) and commercial ginseng

LATIN NAME: Unknown (California ginseng)
Panax quinqufolius (Chinese ginseng)

NATIVE PLANT: Yes and no, respectively.

PART USED: Root

USE: For cleansing the liver, strengthening the uterine wall after pregnancy, and treating prostate problems.

PREPARATION: Josephine has obtained Chinese ginseng commercially in several forms: as a boxful of roots, about the size of a big matchbox and containing about 24 roots; powdered in teabags; and, most recently, in the form of a brown crystallized juice extract.

DOSAGE: Dry and pound the root. Drink a teaspoon of the powder in one cup of hot water, or alternatively, in a cup of coffee in the morning.

When she was able to gather ginseng, Josephine would put the root through a chopper, then save the milk that came from it. The milk hardens into a brown crystal. To cleanse the liver, break off a piece of the crystal and suck on it until it dissolves. Repeat daily for about a week.

Commercial producers make the crystallized extract about two or three inches long: *They taper from a quarter of an inch down. We've got to break it.*

To clear up discharge after pregnancy, drink a cup of the tea, using the teabag form, twice a day for a month. For prostate problems, take twice a day for a good three to four weeks: *It isn't going to hurt you no matter how long you take it.*
White ginseng is a small plant, less than six inches high, with roots about three feet long. Josephine has unsuccessfully tried to grow ginseng in her yard. She suspects that the soil type is integral to success, with a high iron content required. Ginseng sap is available commercially. It comes out of British Columbia.

Once health food stores opened and demand increased, excessive harvesting entirely eliminated ginseng locally. Josephine once gathered ginseng around home sites at a camp where Chinese workers had lived. About unethical herbalists, Josephine laments: *They don't leave anything for seed.*

Like red raspberry, ginseng strengthens the uterine wall: *You use it after pregnancy... Another one that's related to the ginseng family is what we call bearberries. Spikenard. That's a good one for douches.*

See also: raspberry, red and spikenard.

Goldenseal

LATIN NAME: *Hydrastis canadensis*

NATIVE PLANT: No

PART USED: Root

USE: This herb serves as a type of cure-all. Goldenseal cleanses the blood, is effective for sore throats, colitis, ulcers, and expelling parasites from the system: *If you have colitis or ulcers, it's a good healer. It cleanses your liver. If there's an herb that turns yellow when you fix it, it's good for a cleanser. Like the Oregon grape root. We take that for a blood purifier. And the dock will turn pale yellow when you fix the root part.* Take goldenseal for cleansing of the liver and pancreas. Cancer and HIV/AIDS patients especially benefit from this kind of cleansing. Also used to treat worms in dogs.

PREPARATION: Put in double ought capsules. Add peppermint or spearmint to the blood purifier for taste. For dogs with worms, roll a double ought capsule up inside hamburger. For preparation details of gargle for sore throat, see the section on gargles in "Types of Medicinals."

DOSAGE: Many people are allergic to goldenseal. Don't exceed the prescribed dosages. Taking a lot doesn't help: *It's a bitter thing. I always put it in big [double ought] capsules. You can't take goldenseal too long. I'd say maybe for two days, then quit. It heals right away. You can get it in liquid form in health food stores, but then only use about one or two drops in a cup of water. You'll still taste the bitter. If you've got a sore throat, gargle with it maybe two or three times a day, and* [the sore throat is] *gone.* Take two capsules per day, one each in the morning and evening for two days. Drink in liquid form twice a day for two days. Drink a quart once a day for two days to cleanse the lining of the intestine and remove dead skin. For worms, give dogs one capsule, wait two days, and give them another. Wait another two days, then give dogs a final capsule. Three capsules should be enough.

Goldenseal is something that came in recently. We didn't have it here until I met with Doctor Bear up in Montana. I can't remember which city he was from any more, but he was a feather doctor. He went around and tapped you all over with a feather. I don't know what that feather does. It'll come down to wherever your ailment is. You stand in a little circle when he's tapping you with the feather.

Josephine met Doctor Bear in the 1960s: *In the '60s and '70s I went to a lot of meetings and gatherings. That's when all the diseases came out. All these diseases they've got nowadays. Stuff that's caused by people experimenting with drugs.*

He's the one introduced us to the goldenseal. There used to be a few plants [growing locally], *but I think people brought it in. I get it up north. While he was alive, he used to gather it and send it, or bring it down when he came.*

Josephine once tried goldenseal as a cleanser for a patient with hepatitis, but the patient turned out to be allergic, and vomited it up. Other patients use it with no ill effect.

Grindelia is also good for treating parasites in the system.

See also: dock, yellow, grindelia, and Oregon grape root.

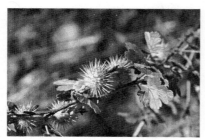

Gooseberry. Photo by Beverly Ortiz

Gooseberry

KARUK NAME: axráttip (Sierra gooseberry, *R. roezlii*) ["gooseberry-bush"]

LATIN NAME: *Ribes roezlii* var. *cruentum*

NATIVE PLANT: Yes

PART USED: To dissolve kidney stones, and, more rarely, gall stones, use the whole plant except the root, including the stems, flowers, leaves, and berries when present. Use the berries for food.

USE: Dissolves kidney stones: *The gooseberry has that acid in it that'll eat the* [calcium deposit of the] *stone up.* Dissolves gravel in the bladder. Breaks up gall stones. Eat the berries raw, and make into pie.

PREPARATION: For medicinal purposes, chop up the plant into inch pieces and steep by the quart. Between uses, store in the refrigerator.

Eat gooseberries raw or make them into pie. For preparation details, see the subsection on gooseberries in the fruit section of "Native Plant Foods."

DOSAGE: Steep half a cup in a quart of hot water. Take for a minimum of two cups per day, morning and evening, up to three cups per day, but no more.

Gooseberry dissolves kidney stones and gravel in the bladder in about two or three days. In contrast, horsetail must be taken for four or five weeks to achieve the same end. To break up gall stones gooseberry tea requires more than six weeks.

osephine's family used the relatively high-elevation mountain gooseberry: *The one at higher elevation didn't have that tough skin on the outside, like the ones down low. We used to put them between two flat rocks and roll it to break all the stickers down. We'd just pop it in our mouth.*

When Josephine was growing up, gooseberry bushes were covered with fruit, and she helped her paternal grandmother gather them for pie. *We used to see lizards under the tree eating it. And squirrels... There used to be a lot of gooseberries in those days, but now you hardly see any... I haven't seen any to eat for years...*

See also: horsetail.

Gotu kola

LATIN NAME: *Centella asiatica*

NATIVE PLANT: No

PART USED: Unknown. Commercially chopped.

USE: Primarily used for memory loss. Reduces blood pressure. Used, as well, to calm hyper children.

PREPARATION: Steep as a tea.

DOSAGE: Use about three quarters of a teaspoon to one cup of hot water. Drink once in the morning and once in the evening. Take for one week, then wait two weeks, and take again, as needed.

Josephine learned about gotu kola from the Chinese boys she worked with years ago. It has never grown locally.

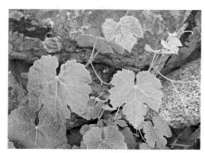

Wild grape. Photo by Jennifer Kalt.

Grape, wild

LATIN NAME: *Vitus californicus*

NATIVE PLANT: Yes

PART USED: Sap

USE: For gout. To prevent hair loss.

PREPARATION: Cut stem in the spring, and let the sap run into a jar.

DOSAGE: For gout, take one teaspoon per day for four or five days, then quit. For hair loss, massage the sap into the scalp two to three times per day for two weeks, thereby aiding in circulation to the scalp area.

Years ago men who worked in the mines wore gumboots. They got gout due to dampness in their feet. It's a condition that comes and goes.

See also: sarsaparilla.

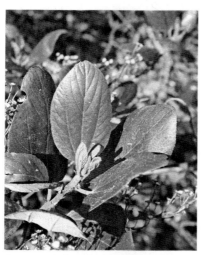

Greasewood. Photo by Jennifer Kalt.

Greasewood (buckbrush)

aka buckthorn and snowbrush, although Josephine doesn't use these common names; rather, she considers buckthorn the *"scientific name."*

KARUK NAME: uyhúrurip

LATIN NAME: *Ceanothus velutinus*

NATIVE PLANT: Yes

PART USED: Sap

USE: Shrinks varicose veins.

PREPARATION: Scrape and peel back the bark. You'll see a *"slimy jell"* (sap) against the stem. Scrape the sap into a glass jar and refrigerate. Poultice this on varicose veins externally.

Dip bandage in a small amount of sterile water, then squeeze it out, so only enough remains to keep the bandage moist. Put the sap on the bandage and apply to varicose vein. Alternatively, rub the sap on varicose vein, poultice with a cloth wrapping, then cover with plastic to retain moisture.

DOSAGE: Keep poultice in place for two days, then remove it. If not healed, apply a new poultice. For bad cases, varicose veins can take a week to heal.

Josephine learned about greasewood in the 1940s and 1950s from an *"old timer"* in the area she got to talking with about it. It grows near Redding.

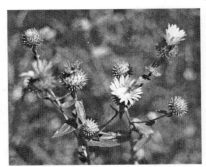

Grindelia. Photo by Beverly Ortiz.

Grindelia (gum plant)

Josephine uses these names interchangeably.

LATIN NAME: *Grindelia hirsutula*

NATIVE PLANT: Yes

PART USED: Tops, including the flowers.

USE: For settling the stomach. *Anyone with stomach trouble can take it.* Grindelia's especially helpful for HIV/AIDS and cancer patients. Cleans the stomach lining and intestine walls. Expels internal parasites.

PREPARATION: Pick when the leaves are green. Steep as a tea. Drink before taking wild peach as a cancer treatment.

DOSAGE: Steep about half a cup of grindelia in a quart of hot water. This will keep in the refrigerator for two days, and may be reheated as needed.

Drink a cup thirty minutes before eating. Take grindelia on the days the stomach is really upset. For cancer patients, drink about half a cup, then wait half an hour and drink the wild peach. Grindelia settles the stomach so the wild peach will stay down. Take both for about three weeks. After taking grindelia for two to three days, the stomach lining, when expelled, will look like coconut. *All of the sudden you'll get really sick, and you'll vomit what will look like a bunch of hair. This is fevers of the cancer coming out. A lot of patients will only take it just so long, then quit. They get scared when they get sick. But you take it three weeks, then you stop for a week or two, then you take it again.*

For treating internal parasites, take half a cup twice a day for two days.

Chinese miners planted this plant in the local area. Josephine used to obtain grindelia for Grandma Flora Jones, a Wintun healer, as well as purple Jimson weed.

See also: peach, wild.

Hawthorn

LATIN NAME: Unknown. *Crataegus oxyacanthus* (English hawthorn). *C. mouogyna* is sold as hawthorn in health food stores.

NATIVE PLANT: No. Planted in the Hoopa Valley. A native hawthorn (*C. douglasii*) grows above 700 meters to the east of Hoopa, but isn't likely to grow in the valley.

PART USED: Bark

USE: Hawthorn mildly dilates coronary blood vessels and strengthens the heart muscle. It's useful for arteriosclerosis.

PREPARATION: Skin the bark off, then dry it.

DOSAGE: Experience has taught Josephine the proper dosage: *I have them try a quarter of a cup first. If they're allergic to it, they'll know right away. They'll just vomit it right up.*

We never had hawthorn here. We had to get it from elsewhere. I don't remember just how it came here. We used to gather the berries on the ground, and the bark. There's two different kinds. We use the one that's more like a shrub than a tree.

Josephine doesn't recall when she first became aware of hawthorn's benefits for people with heart trouble.

See also: choke-cherry and dogwood.

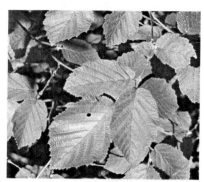
Hazel. Photo by Jennifer Kalt.

Hazel

LATIN NAME: *Corylus cornuta* var. *californica*

NATIVE PLANT: Yes

PART USED: Nuts

USE: Food

PREPARATION: Gather nuts in the fall. For gathering and processing details, see the subsection on hazelnuts in the nuts section of "Native Plant Foods."

DOSAGE: N/A

Josephine has seen crows eat the nuts, and squirrels crawl up on the bushes to get at them. The shoots of this plant are also used for basketry.

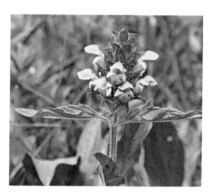
Heal-all. Photo by Jennifer Kalt.

Heal-all (self heal)

LATIN NAME: *Prunella vulgaris*

NATIVE PLANT: No

PART USED: Stem and leaves for most purposes. Pick the flowers off. Root and upper part of the plant, including the flower if in blossom, in salves

USE: Heal-all is a good blood purifier. It's taken as a tea for fits and convulsions. It's used with Knox gelatin for bleeding ulcers. It's chewed for bleeding gums. It's used in a salve with coltsfoot, wormwood, and Johnny-jump-up (violet) for sores that don't heal (ulcerated sores, external cancerous sores, bedsores). It's used with choke-cherry and mountain balm to make a cough, asthma, bronchitis, whooping cough, and pneumonia syrup.

PREPARATION: Use heal-all fresh or hang it upside down to dry, then store it in jars. The tea and its gelled version will keep in the refrigerator for several days.

For a blood purifier, and fits and convulsions, steep as a tea. For bleeding ulcers, make tea, then add Knox gelatin: *If you can't get the gel out of the Solomon seal for bleeding ulcers, then I take plain old gelatin and mix it in with the heal-all when you drink it. The gelatin seals the tissue for ulcers, and the heal-all will heal. You'd put maybe a good heaping teaspoonful of gelatin in a measuring cup of water with your self heal.* First make the tea, then stir in enough gelatin for jelling to occur.

For preparation details of salve and syrup, see the sections on salves and cough syrups in "Types of Medicinals."

DOSAGE: Use the standard teaspoon to one cup of hot water. Because of its qualities as a blood purifier, Josephine finds heal-all useful in all her herbal remedies: *I'll probably put in a tablespoonful if I'm brewing up a batch of medicine for somebody. Maybe a quart. You could call it a quart. Or a gallon.*

For a blood purifier, Josephine recommends drinking two cups of heal-all a day, once in the morning, and once in the evening, for six weeks in spring and fall.

When you feel a fit or convulsion coming on, one cupful of the tea is enough to prevent it.

For bleeding ulcers, take a good spoonful to half a cup a day until healed in about a week.

For people that have gum sores—bleeding gums—we chew the raw plant. We just pick it and chew it a couple of times a day. If using dry, soak heal-all in cold water until it becomes chewable.

Apply salve periodically until healed. Take syrup as needed.

As one walks through the gate into Josephine's Hoopa Valley yard, heal-all is visible in the plant beds that line either side of the pathway, where Josephine broadcast the seeds some years back. Although heal-all dies back during the winter, it's often possible to find some fresh leaves close to the ground late into the season. *If we get a good frost, then you don't see it.*

When Josephine was a child, heal-all was used as a blood purifier in the spring and fall: *We'd take it as a blood purifier. In the fall it kind of immunes you from catching flu and cold. Everybody did it. All the old folks. We use the peppernuts same way. You roast the peppernut and eat four or five a day during the winter months. That keeps you from catching a cold by building up your immune system. I keep a jar of peppernuts around.*

See also: coltsfoot, Johnny-jump-up, wormwood, peppernuts, and mistletoe.

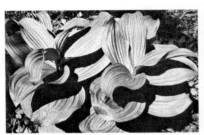

False hellebore (Veratrum sp.).
Photo by Beverly Ortiz.

Hellebore, false

LATIN NAME: Probably *Veratrum viride*

NATIVE PLANT: Yes

PART USED: Root. The root of false hellebore looks like "*a big, dirty, old mop.*"

USE: Use for treating pneumonia. Take it for strep throat, whether you feel sick or not.

PREPARATION: Pull up one whole stem and collect the roots. Purchase commercially from Canada and Alaska.

DOSAGE: Let an inch-length of the root dissolve between the cheek and gums until all that remains is the wire-like center of the root. Don't take too much, as "*a funny feeling*" on the back of your tongue can occur, akin to the paralyzing feel of a black widow bite.

The coastal Indians from British Columbia north into Alaska used false hellebro, which grows in high-elevation swampy areas. Its leaves, with their wide veins, and its stalk, with its bushy flower, cause false hellebro to resemble a large false Solomon seal.

Hops

LATIN NAME: *Humulus lupulus*

NATIVE PLANT: No, but cultivated locally

PART USED: Pollen

USE: Insomnia or restlessness due to shock. Good for the liver. Decreases the desire for alcohol. *Alfalfa tea is another one you can take to help you not drink alcohol.*

PREPARATION: *Hop flowers have a lot of yellow powder... We'd pick them, shake the pollen into a jar, and save it.* When picking the flowers, be careful not to touch the vine, as hops have barbs that will cause the skin to welt.

DOSAGE: Take a handful or so of pollen, soak it in water and drink cold: *It isn't going to hurt you no matter how much you take.*

When Josephine was growing up, everybody in the area planted hops, letting them vine up lengths of string. Hops were used for porch shade, and put over windows to block the summertime sun. The use of hops in beer making was a commercial rather than domestic activity.

See also: alfalfa.

Horehound

LATIN NAME: *Marrubium vulgare*

NATIVE PLANT: No, but locally naturalized

PART USED: Primarily the stem and leaves, but the flowers may be included when in bloom.

USE: Colds, breaking a fever, jaundice, lung trouble (asthma), sore throat, coughs, and the croup.

PREPARATION: Use fresh or dried. To break a fever, drink horehound hot. The tea is also good for colds, jaundice, lung trouble (asthma), sore throat, coughs, and the croup.

For sore throat, make a strong tea to gargle with. For preparation and use details, see the section on gargles in "Types of Medicinals."

For coughs, make a syrup with horehound and mountain balm. Use brandy or rum in the syrup to preserve it. For whooping cough, add a little marijuana to the syrup. For croup, made a syrup solely with horehound. For preparation and use details of syrups, see the section on cough syrups in "Types of Medicinals."

DOSAGE: For the tea, Josephine steeps a teaspoonful of horehound in one cup of hot water. The number of dosages depends on need. For breaking a fever, take every four hours. For jaundice, take two times a day for a week or so. For asthma, drink as much as you can handle during an attack. Alternatively, use the syrup for asthma.

For croup, take as a syrup or tea every four hours until cured.

[Horehound] *used to grow on all the river bars. I had one [plant] growing out here [in my front yard] and one in the back. We had to use it all when we had the big fires. Everybody's lungs were all clogged up from* [the smoke]. Josephine refers, here, to the Meagram Fire of 1999, which lasted for about three months and burned some 125,000 acres. She prescribed a syrup of horehound, mountain balm, and marijuana to ease the stuffed-up effect of smoke in the lungs of firefighters and cook camp personnel.

You can buy horehound candy in the stores. My dad always bought it. He always brought us home horehound candies. That was his big thing, I guess, to keep us from catching cold [laughs].

Ho shou wu

LATIN NAME: Unknown. *Polygonum multifloum* is sold commercially as ho shou wu.

NATIVE PLANT: No

PART USED: Root and leaves.

USE: Similar to ginseng, this herb has restorative powers, helping to build up the immune system. It's used for longevity, tumors, piles, menstrual problems, liver, spleen, constipation and insomnia.

PREPARATION: Ho shou wu may be used to treat all the listed conditions in tea, tonic, or cold, liquid form: *It's made into a tea. A long time ago, they used to grind it all up, and make it into a patty. Then, when you have to use it, you break off a little piece, and put it in a tea. It'll dissolve.*

We'd make it into a tonic.[30] *You put boiling water in it, then a little bit of alcohol in it to keep it from spoiling. You mix other herbs with it, too. With ginseng, you can put ginger root in it.* Ginger root refers here to wild ginger root, which is in the same family of plants as ho shou wu. To make the tonic, barely cover an equal amount of ho shou wu, wild ginger root and ginseng with water, then simmer. Strain out the herbs. Add a little honey for taste before the tonic cools. After it cools, add alcohol (brandy or rum) as a preservative.

In patty (cake) form, ho shou wu was referred to as "cow cake." To form the patty (cake), first scrub the roots and break up the plant. Mash the root and leaves with a hammer, then dry it on a piece of wax paper. Break off a piece, as needed, for tea.

Today ho shou wu comes in a box. Boil a quart of water, to sterilize the tea water, then let the water cool. Dissolve a half-inch by three-quarter-inch piece of ho shou wu in the cold water.

DOSAGE: Josephine drinks a quart of the ho shou wu that comes in a box within two days. Since the tea should be fresh, when consumed, it may be necessary to quarter the amount of herb and water.

For longevity, take in any amount. For tumors, take one or two cups a day for as many days as you wish. For piles, take two cups a day for as many days as the condition exists. For menstrual problems, begin taking two days before your period, when feeling bloated, and continue until your period ends. For the liver and spleen, drink two cups per day. Make fresh as often as you can, and take for at least four to six weeks to cleanse. Make fresh as often as you can. For constipation, drink two cups a day for two days. For insomnia, drink some before you go to bed.

This plant is a "cousin" to ginseng: *It's in the ginseng family. It doesn't grow in here at all. It grows in British Columbia... I found it there.* Josephine learned about this plant from the sons of a Chinese herbalist with whom she used to gather herbs when she was young. *They always called it ho shou wu.*

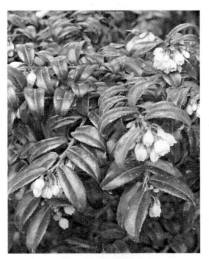

Huckleberry. Photo by Jennifer Kalt.

Huckleberry

KARUK NAME: purith'ippan ["huckleberry-bush"] [-*ip*: "-bush"]

LATIN NAME: *Vaccinium ovatum*

NATIVE PLANT: Yes

PART USED: New leaves.

USE: Medicinal: Diabetes, insomnia. Food: Fresh, canned, jam, duff, fried pies, and steam pudding.

PREPARATION: For a medicinal tea, harvest the fresh growth, which is lighter green, then dry the leaves and steep them in hot water. Eat berries fresh. For information about gathering, cleaning, drying and storing the berries, see the fruit section in "Native Plant Foods," and the subsection on huckleberries. For information about huckleberry food preparation, see the subsections on canned fruit, and jams and jellies, in the cooking with fruit section of "Native Plant Foods"; and the subsections on duff, fried pies, and steam pudding, in the pastry section of "Native Plant Foods."

DOSAGE: Use the standard teaspoon of leaves to one cup of water. A person can take as much of this herb as they wish without any ill effect, although, since huckleberry tea induces sleep, patients will sleep all day if they take too much.

For diabetes, take one cup two to three times a day for the rest of your life: *I think the reason it helps diabetes is because it helps you relax.*

When Josephine was growing up, there was no name for diabetes, although the old people took huckleberry tea to ease the symptoms, as well as for insomnia. Josephine thinks that what the locals called dropsy in the old days was actually diabetes.

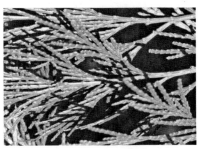

Incense cedar. Photo by Jennifer Kalt.

Incense cedar

KARUK NAME: chuneexneeyâach

LATIN NAME: *Calocedrus decurrens*

NATIVE PLANT: Yes

PART USED: Boughs

USE: Cleansing the scene of a death.

PREPARATION: When somebody close to you has died out-of-doors, spread incense cedar ashes over any blood or hair, and brush the site off with incense cedar greenery. If clothing or other personal effects remain, burn these at the river bar, where rocks, rather than sand, have built up along the river.

DOSAGE: N/A

This is how Josephine handles out-of-doors deaths. Others have alternative methods, such as hanging the clothing from a stick, and starting a hot drift-wood- and cedar-bough fire on the ground beneath. At times, people burn all the personal effects of the deceased, including baskets, in a metal trash bin.

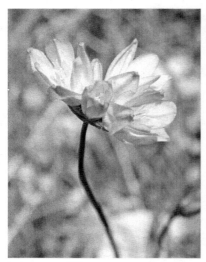

Indian potato (*Dichelostemma capitatum*).
Photo by Jennifer Kalt.

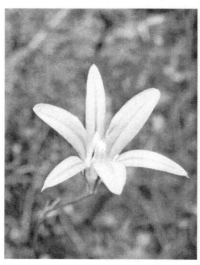

Indian potato (*Tritelia laxa*).
Photo by Jennifer Kalt.

Indian potato (blue camas)

LATIN NAME: *Dichelostemma capitatum*

NATIVE PLANT: Yes

PART USED: Corms

USE: Food

PREPARATION: *The only time you can get them is when they bloom. Eat raw. Cook in stews.*

DOSAGE: N/A

Indian potatoes, some inch to an inch-and-a-half long, grew in profusion outside the fence and back garden at the Old Home Place. They also grew near the school. Each "*potato*" (corm) supported a cluster of perhaps six or seven little, purple blossoms, about an inch to an inch-and-a-quarter across. When the blossoms dropped off, a seed pod that looked like a little green potato stood out on top.

Josephine's father created a specialized, T-shaped digging tool out of about twenty inches of galvanized pipe, about half an inch in diameter. After heating the pipe in a forge, he'd flatten it on one end to make a spoon-shaped digging instrument, which easily dug the bulbs, which could be found about two inches or so beneath the ground's surface.

When Josephine was growing up, she and her siblings dug Indian potatoes and ate them raw "*just to be doing something.*" This plant grew along the trails between the Old Home Place and school. Today, the gophers get to the Indian potatoes before people can. A lot of Indian potatoes once grew on a flat, but the gophers destroyed this patch. Josephine obtains hers in a local field.

Of the two species of *Brodiaea* that grow in the Klamath Range Floristic Province; four species of *Dichelostemma*; and six species of *Triteleia*, the following have purple blossoms: *Brodiaea coronaria*, *B. elegans*, *Dichelostemma capitatum*,[31] *D. congestum*,[32] *D. multilflorum*,[33] *Triteleia bridgesii*, and *T. laxa*.[34] In 1939, Karuk cultural consultants described the cooking of *Triteleia laxa*:

> They dig a pit, line it with rocks, and build a fire in it. As soon as the fire has burned out, the pit is cleaned of ashes and the cleaned bulbs are put in on a mat of fresh maple leaves, then another mat of maple leaves is laid over them. Madrone leaves are put on top of this, then hot rocks. The hot rocks are covered with earth and on this a fire is built. The bulbs are eaten the next day when the pit is opened. (Schenck and Gifford 1952:380)

Indian root (angelica)

KARUK NAME: kuríthxiit (California angelica, *A. tomentosa*, before it flowers) [-*xíit*: "new"] *mahimkaanva* (California angelica, *A. tomentosa*, after it flowers) ["uphill-greens"]

LATIN NAME: *Angelica tomentosa*

NATIVE PLANT: Yes

PART USED: Root for medicinal purposes; leaves and stems for food.

USE: Blood purifier. Used for sour stomach, gas, heartburn, colic, and colds. Colic results when "*babies get too much wind.*" By relieving gas, you prevent heartburn. Also used for food.

PREPARATION: For blood purifier, steep the root in hot water for tea. If dry, first soak the root in warm water for about an hour.

For sour stomach, gas, and colic, steep fresh or dried root as a tea. Alternatively, chew the root.

For food, dry the stems (with leaves) when they're about six inches high, prior to blossoming, and use in stews and soups instead of celery.

Chew the tender, inside portion of the fresh root for enjoyment. *A lot of them would eat it.* [....] *We used to chew it just to be chewing it.*

DOSAGE: Depending on the root's size, it will need to be cut up. Put a small, slender root, about finger-sized, in the jar, then steep in the standard manner, covered while hot. Store in the refrigerator. Josephine will drink the tea *"just to be doing it."*

Since angelica isn't plentiful, and thus Josephine must go a distance to get it, she only takes it for about two days, twice a day, for its blood purifying qualities. More often, instead, she takes Oregon grape in the spring for the full six weeks.

For sour stomach, gas, and colic, steep a teaspoon of dried or fresh root in one cup of water. For sour stomach and gas, drink one half to a full cup one time. For colic, dispense about one-half teaspoonful. Alternatively, chew angelica for sour stomach and gas.

Due to its scarcity, Josephine rarely takes angelica for colds: *When you feel a cold coming on, mix up the yerba buena, and drink about two or three hot cups of that to stop it.* Josephine once tried growing angelica from seed, but was unsuccessful. She has seen it growing in shale and other bedrock, and supposes it needs a lot of iron to grow. She mused: *I should try throwing a bucket of nails in the ground.*

See also: yerba buena.

Iris (string iris)

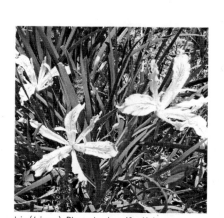

Iris (*Iris* sp.). Photo by Jennifer Kalt.

LATIN NAME: *Iris macrosiphon*

NATIVE PLANT: Yes

PART USED: Leaf

USE: Cordage

PREPARATION: Gather selected leaves in the spring. Cut them down low. Put them on any flat surface, such as a board, then pound them with a curve-bottomed rock, and peel out the fibers. Each leaf yields about two usable fibers. Twist the fibers into a two-ply string by rolling them against the thigh away from the body. When they rolled the fibers, the *"old ladies"* used to get dark-green marks on their thighs, hands and fingernails from the chlorophyll-laden juice: *They get kind of brown looking.* As needed, splice in more fibers, leaving the cord slack while you lay the new pieces in. Tuck the new ends between the old ends, so they won't show, and the cord will be smooth: *You can splice in the little ones.* Wrap the finished string around a wooden shuttle.

DOSAGE: N/A

Josephine learned how to make iris cordage from Anthony Risling (Yurok, Karuk, member of the Hoopa Valley Tribe). *Anthony and I used to go and teach it in the school.* For another description of Anthony's technique, see Ortiz (1999/2000).

Jimson weed (with purple stem)

LATIN NAME: Probably *Datura wrightii*, but may be *Datura stramonium*

NATIVE PLANT: Native, but not local. The flowers look nearly identical on all species of jimson weed. Josephine gathers a species with a purple stem: *The ones with the purple stem are kind of bushy and stay close to the ground...*

PART USED: Stem and leaves.

USE: Use with wormwood for easing the pain of severely diabetic feet that do not have sores. The wormwood eases swelling. When pain isn't present, the use of Jimson weed is unnecessary.

PREPARATION: *For ones that have diabetes really bad, where the feet turn color, we use wormwood and Jimson weed for soaking... I think it kills the pain in your feet.* Soak feet in a bubble spa to aid circulation in swollen feet and legs. For preparation details, see the section on soaks in "Types of Medicinals."

DOSAGE: Use as much wormwood as you wish, but only a little bit of Jimson weed. *When you soak your feet in Jimson weed, it's going to absorb into your skin, so you can't do it too long... We do it for about twenty minutes... If they have a lot of sores, we don't use that one. We just use plain wormwood. But if their skin's not broken, then we can use a lot of the Jimson weed...* Use the soak with wormwood and Jimson weed for two to three days. Continue using wormwood on subsequent days for swelling, every day as needed, for as long as patient can manage. *The longer they can keep their feet in the better.*

When Josephine was growing up, there was no name for diabetes. Josephine thinks that what the locals called dropsy in the old days was actually diabetes.

See also: wormwood.

Johnny jump-up. Photo by Jennifer Kalt

Johnny jump-up (violet, wild pansy), garden violet

LATIN NAME: *Viola ocellata* and *Viola* sp. respectively. A pressed plant specimen labeled by Josephine as garden violet has *Viola odorata* as the Latin name, although this identification has not been confirmed.

NATIVE PLANT: Yes and no, respectively.

PART USED: Whole plant for reducing fevers. Leaves for tea and wash. Root and top of plant, including the flowers, if in bloom, for salve.

USE: For reducing fevers and headaches, and killing the pain of sores that don't heal, such as ulcerated sores and bedsores. This plant has the same effect as aspirin, relieving pain. It will even work on a hurt elbow.

PREPARATION: Steep whole plant as tea for reducing fevers. Steep leaves for headaches. Make wash out of a strong tea for cleansing sores that don't heal. For preparation details, see the section on washes in "Types of Medicinals." Make salve with violet only if feeling pain. Make salve with coltsfoot, heal-all, and wormwood for treating sores that don't heal (skin sores, bedsores, and external cancerous sores). Make salve with coltsfoot, plantain, and wormwood for treating boils, ulcerated sores, and skin diseases, such as psoriasis, scabies, mange, and ringworm). For preparation details of salves, see the section on salves in "Types of Medicinals."

DOSAGE: Make tea using the standard teaspoon to one cup of hot water. For reducing fevers, take tea every two hours until the fever breaks. For headache, take half a cup to start. If no relief, take a little more. Take every two hours until the headache stops.

For wash, apply as much as you can while the wash is still warm.

Apply salve periodically until healed.

Josephine learned about Johnny-jump-up from the "*old people.*" She has been successful planting it in her yard: *In my yard mine stay good all year around.*

Both Johnny-jump-up and garden violet can be used for teas, washes, and salves. The washes and salves work equally well for sores that don't heal.

See also: coltsfoot, heal-all, elderberry, Johnny-jump-up, plantain, ribbed, and wormwood.

Juniper

LATIN NAME: *Juniperus communis.* According to botanist Bert Johnson, a pressed plant specimen labeled by Josephine as *Juniperus communis* is probably *J. occidentalis* or *J. osteasperma*, indicating that Josephine likely does not distinguish between the juniper species she uses medicinally.

NATIVE PLANT: Yes

PART USED: "*Berries*" (fleshy cone).

USE: Used for kidney and bladder problems related to the pancreas and adrenal glands. Also used for dropsy and prostate: *It's hard on your kidneys, but it's supposed to be a good medicine for it, too, if you don't take too much. And it's good for bladder problems.*

PREPARATION: *If it's fresh, we can put it in, pour hot water on it, and just let it steep. Then we have to strain the water to get the pitch out. But lots of it stays in. You can taste it.* When dry, soak the berries, pour the water off, and then re-steep: *You've got to soak it quite a while.*

DOSAGE: Do not take if pregnant, as juniper will abort. Josephine has her patients take about half a cup, brewed as a tea, twice a day for no more than three days. She takes care to give such small doses, because, given this plant's toxic qualities, "*You can kill somebody.*"

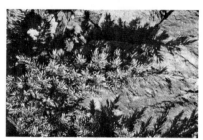

Juniper. Photo courtesy East Bay Regional Park District Botanic Garden.

Juniper leaves. Photo courtesy East Bay Regional Park District Botanic Garden.

Since juniper berries were hard to get locally, they were traded back and forth. A long time ago that's how we got them. Josephine developed her own gathering places. She knew a beader from Pocatello, Idaho, in the 1960s and 1970s, or earlier, who, although she didn't use juniper in her own beadwork, told Josephine where she could obtain the "*berries*" (fleshy cones) on the outskirts of Pocatello. At the time, both women followed the powwow circuit, setting up booths, and they would periodically meet up: *[T]hat's when we learned how to really go after juniper berries and get them.* The trees grow right out of the boulders at this locale, becoming stunted in the process. Since it was necessary to jump from boulder to boulder to access the berries, Josephine always brought at least one helper: *Most of the time the younger ones have to go get it.*

I always went up to McArthur and Burney around hunting season time to get it. We can pick them and dry them. When we use them for medicines, we pick the hull, too, and let it dry, because the pitch and turpentine is in that.

We collect the juniper seeds for our regalia... To process the seeds for use on regalia, boil the cones to remove the scales ("*hull*"), then reboil and strain the seeds three times to remove the pitch and turpentine residue: *We always soak it, pour off that same water that we soak it in, then bring it to a boil, and pour it back off.* Next, put a hole through the seed: *If you get them fresh, you can poke a hole through them with a needle. But if they're dry...you've got to drill them. They always say you put them on an ant hill. That's an old woman's tale. The ants'll eat out the inside. Put a hole in it for you* [laughs]... *That's what they used to tell us a long time ago, but I never found an ant hill with any in it* [laughs].

A long time ago, the old people took it for birth control. They knew when to brew it up and drink it. Each month they'd do that... They picked the berries and dried them, and to prevent getting pregnant, they'd take the tea before their period and for five days afterward. Josephine recommends against this, since young women can kill themselves by taking juniper berry tea for birth control.

When Josephine was growing up, there was no name for diabetes. Josephine thinks that what the locals called dropsy in the old days was actually diabetes.

Knotweed

LATIN NAME: *Polygonum arenastrum*

NATIVE PLANT: Yes

PART USED: Top of the whole plant, including the tiny flowers, when present.

USE: Back pain.

PREPARATION: Use fresh or dried. Steep as a tea.

DOSAGE: Use a teaspoon to one cup of hot water. Take some three cups spread throughout the day until the back pain is gone.

This plant has the same medicinal use as lady's thumb (Polygonum *persicaria*).

See also: lady's thumb.

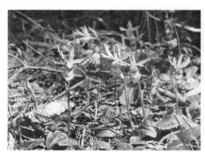

Pink lady slipper. Photo courtesy East Bay Regional Park District Botanic Garden.

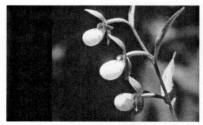

White lady slipper, flower detail. Photo courtesy East Bay Regional Park District Botanic Garden.

Lady slipper, pink and white

KARUK NAME: pihneefyukkúkkuh (*C. californicum*) ["coyote-shoes"]

LATIN NAME: *Calypso bulbosa* (pink lady slipper)
Cypripedium californicum (white lady slipper)

NATIVE PLANT: Yes

PART USED: Bulb

USE: Use for convulsions and epilepsy, in combination with mistletoe.

PREPARATION: Gather the peanut-sized bulb in the spring. Chop up the bulb, then dry it. Always use with "*not too much*" mistletoe.

DOSAGE: Dosage withheld due to dangerous qualities of mistletoe: *You've got to be careful with the mistletoe. Mistletoe can be poisonous, and it will also abort.*

See also: mistletoe.

Lady's thumb (joint weed)

LATIN NAME: *Polygonum persicaria*

NATIVE PLANT: Yes

PART USED: Top of the whole plant, including the tiny flowers, when present.

USE: Back pain: *I think that's why it's called joint weed. The vertebrae fit together.*

PREPARATION: Use fresh or dried. Steep as a tea.

DOSAGE: Use a teaspoon of lady's thumb to one cup of hot water. Take some three cups spread throughout the day until the back pain is gone.

This flat-laying plant grows through cement. Josephine learned about it from the Chinese doctor in Red Bluff whose sons she worked with. It has the same medicinal use as knotweed (*Polygonum arenastrum*).

See also: knotweed.

Lemon grass

LATIN NAME: *Cymbopogon hirtus. C. citrates* and *C. flexuous* are sold commercially as lemon grass.

NATIVE PLANT: No

PART USED: Straw

USE: Childhood drink. Non-medicinal tea.

PREPARATION: Steep as a tea.

DOSAGE: N/A

Josephine was first introduced to this plant at age seven or eight. It served as the basis of a childhood drink she and her siblings used to experiment with: *We used to try all kinds of things.*

The Raleigh man brought lemon grass to the Somes Bar area. It grows around Monterey and Santa Cruz.

When dry, this plant has the appearance of oat straw. Josephine used to obtain hers from friends in Monterey, who sent it up, and, during summertime visits, delivered it in person.

Lemon mint (citronella)

Josephine uses the name lemon mint and citronella interchangeably.

LATIN NAME: Probably *Melissa officinalis*

NATIVE PLANT: Unknown

PART USED: Top of plant.

USE: Mosquito repellent.

PREPARATION: Dry the plant, break it up and store it. For repelling mosquitoes, make a candle. Boil two cups of water with one cup of lemon mint plant tops and simmer until most of the water evaporates. Strain, retaining the plant material. Mix this with melted beeswax and add a wick.

DOSAGE: N/A

In early times, women put sprigs of this plant in their hair because of its fresh, sweet fragrance.

See also: ginger.

Licorice fern

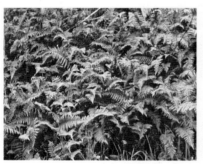

Licorice fern. Photo courtesy East Bay Regional Park District Botanic Garden.

LATIN NAME: *Polypodium glycyrrhiza*

NATIVE PLANT: Yes

PART USED: Root. *It's kind of a succulent thing.*

USE: Used for its sweet flavor, not medicinally.

PREPARATION: Wash the root, which lacks a bark, suck on it, then drink cold water: *We'd stop and drink at the springs along the way home. It gives a sweet taste in your mouth.*

DOSAGE: N/A

This small, six-to-eight inch-long fern grew out of the moss that formed "*up the side*" of oak trees near where Josephine lived as a child. It also grew out of bedrock along mossy creek banks. On their way home from school, Josephine and her siblings would pull the root up through the moss.

Licorice plant

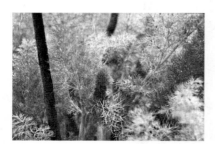

Licorice plant. Photo by Beverly Ortiz.

aka sweet fennel, a common name that Josephine does not use

LATIN NAME: *Foeniculum vulgaris*

NATIVE PLANT: No

PART USED: Top

USE: Used for flavoring medicines that taste poorly.

PREPARATION: N/A

DOSAGE: N/A

Licorice root

LATIN NAME: Unknown

NATIVE PLANT: Yes

PART USED: Top

USE: Used for flavoring.

PREPARATION: Break off about a handful of the plant, place this in a quart of water, then let it sit until the water achieves the desired flavor. A quart or two will last for a couple of days without refrigeration. Alternatively, place a little in water in a Pyrex coffee pot on the back of the woodstove. As desired, pour a little of the now-flavored water out of the pot, add cold water, and drink.

DOSAGE: Make it as strongly-flavored as you like.

When Josephine was growing up, some licorice grew along the children's three-mile route to school. On the way home, Josephine and her siblings would pick some, then suck on the little, long, brown "*buds*" on top. When they arrived at a certain creek and drank the water, the residual licorice flavor made the water taste sweet.

This plant is almost the same as black jack, but it has multiple branches, rather than a single, long seed.

Lily, pond (Indian rhubarb)

KARUK NAME: káaf

LATIN NAME: *Darmera peltata*

NATIVE PLANT: Yes

PART USED: Core of the young shoots.

USE: Food

PREPARATION: *We just pick it, and peel the outer bark off, and eat it. We eat it raw.* Josephine describes the taste as "*odd*" and "*sour.*" *You can peel the new shoots from the blackberry, too, in the spring, when they come up tender, and they taste the same.*

DOSAGE: N/A

When growing up, Josephine and her siblings enjoyed this plant, which they called pond lily: *A lot of times we tried to beat one another to it.* [….] *We'd fight over it.* It grows along creek banks and river bottoms.

See also: blackberry, wild.

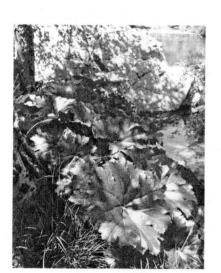

Pond lily. Photo by Sydney Carothers.

Lobelia, blue and cardinal (cardinal flower, red lobelia)

LATIN NAME: *Scutellaria antirrhinoides* (lobelia, blue)

Probably *Mimulus cardinalis* (lobelia, cardinal), based on a pressed plant specimen labeled cardinal flower (red lobelia) by Josephine.

Unknown. The capsules (seed pods) have a distinctive shape, and are the same as those found in a jar Josephine labeled lobelia. Herb stores carry *Lobelia inflata*, which is called Indian tobacco. It grows in the eastern United States and has the same effects as Josephine described.

NATIVE PLANT: Yes and unknown, respectively.

PART USED: Whole plant, including the roots.

USE: Blue lobelia is a strong relaxant. It's useful for stress and the adrenal glands, and emetic in large amounts, and used for angina, epilepsy, ear infection, coughs. It strengthens muscle action. For a weak heart, use with capsicum (cayenne pepper). Cardinal lobelia is used to induce sleep in terminal patients, akin to morphine.

PREPARATION: Make into a tea, or chop until ground, and put into ought capsules. Before Josephine used capsules, she added licorice plant to the tea for taste.

DOSAGE: Withheld, due to its dangerous qualities.

Blue lobelia has purplish blue, trumpet-shaped flowers. Dr. Rickover, and one-time druggist Emmet Smith, used to gather it. The Cardinal, with its little red trumpet flowers, used to grow on rivers, but was taken out by the floods. Both grow as single plants about a foot high: *They look almost alike, and you've got to watch the blooms to see which one it's going to be... The blue lobelia grows in serpentine.*

Since it no longer grows in the local area, Josephine gets most of her lobelia from the Dakotas. *The cardinal lobelia is really powerful, and we don't use that. Only with people who are really sick that we know are on their way out. We give it like they'd give a morphine pill... They'll just sleep. But we can take the blue in medicines in a small amount... It'll relax you... They used to keep lobelia way up high in the cupboard, since they didn't want us [kids] to get a hold of it.*

The blue lobelia will leave a funny feeling in the back of your tongue, like it almost wants to paralyze. I could only open my mouth enough to drink a little water. I had the same feeling when I got bit one time by a black widow... It was inside the gate latch, and it caught me between the fingers.

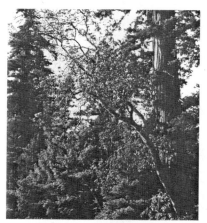

Madrone. Photo by Sydney Carothers.

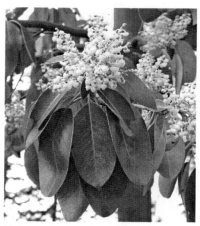

Madrone, detail. Photo by Jennifer Kalt.

Madrone

KARUK NAME: kusrippan (madrone)
kusrippish (madrone berry)

LATIN NAME: *Arbutus menziesii*

NATIVE PLANT: Yes

PART USED: Bark

USE: Diabetes

PREPARATION: Peel off a slab of the bark in the spring, then use a cleaver to chop the bark into small pieces of an inch or less to dry, no more than two by two inches square. Steep as a tea. Use fresh or dry.

DOSAGE: Make one pint using the standard dose of one teaspoon to one cup of hot water three times daily. If needed, take the tea every day to keep blood sugar down.

Although madrone berries are edible, Josephine never ate these. The bark will keep indefinitely. Sometimes people harvest it from cut stumps and give it to Josephine.[35] The bark of madrone will fall off the tree in a thin roll. Josephine and her siblings would create cigarettes out of these bark curls. *We'd all go down by the chicken house* [laughs]. *We had a tree there. We'd sit down and smoke that up.* Inside the roll, they stuffed grass so it would burn.

While Josephine was always aware that the old people gathered this herb, she didn't realize until years later that they used it for diabetes. After she developed diabetes, Josephine began drinking the tea about three times per day for a year. She also ate lots of mushrooms.

Josephine met a Pit River man from the Hat Creek area who told her that his people also used this plant for diabetes, or, as he put it, "blood control."

When Josephine was growing up, there was no name for diabetes. Josephine thinks that what the locals called dropsy in the old days was actually diabetes.

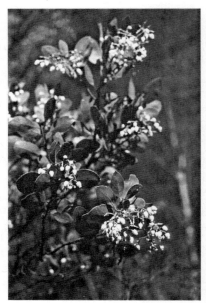

Manzanita (*Manzanita* sp.).
Photo by Beverly Ortiz.

Manzanita

KARUK NAME: fáththip (Parry manzanita, *A. manzanita*)
["manzanita-berry-bush"]
pahav'íppa / fath'uruhsa'ippa (greenleaf manzanita), *A. patula*) [(this species of)] ["manzanita-berry-bush"]

LATIN NAME: *Arctostaphylos canescens* (food) and *A. nevadensis*

NATIVE PLANT: Yes

PART USED: Ashes, bark, stem, leaves, berries, depending on the use.

USE: Used for treating burns and their associated sores. Relieves the itch of poison oak rash. Also used for stomach flu. Made into a sweet drink (cider): *We used to gather the berries a long time ago and make a drink out of it. It's really good.*

PREPARATION: For burns, save the ashes of chopped up manzanita wood burned in the heater stove. Mix some ashes with just enough water to make a paste in your hands. Apply the paste, then "*bandage*" (poultice). For preparation details, see the sections on pastes and poultices in "Types of Medicinals."

For poison oak, boil manzanita leaves with water on the stove as fast as you can. For stomach flu, steep the leaves as a tea.

For preparation details of the sweet drink, see the subsection on manzanita berries in the fruit section of "Native Plant Foods."

DOSAGE: Apply the paste thickly to burns. If you put it on right away, it will remove the sting of the burn, and the burn won't blister. Remove the bandage after two days.

For poison oak itch, the stronger the wash the better. Every time the rash begins to itch, wash with the liquid. Use until the itch is gone.

For stomach flu, use the standard dosage of a teaspoon of leaves to one cup of water. Take three times a day until the stomach settles.

The tannins in manzanita and acorn enable them to heal burns. The following manzanitas grow in the Klamath Ranges: *Arctostaphylos canescens* (hoary manzanita) (subsp. *sonomensis*) with its hairy, 5-10 mm. fruits; *A columbiana* (hairy manzanita) with its "sparsely hairy," 8-11 mm. fruits; *A. glandulosa* (Eastwood's Manzanita) with its hairy to smooth or sticky 6-10 mm. fruits; the uncommon *A. hispidula*, with its 5-7 mm. fruits; *A. klamathensis*, the endemic Klamath manzanita, with its ribbed, 6-7 mm. fruits; *A. nevadensis* (pinemat manzanita), with its glabrous, 6-8 mm. fruits; *A. nortensis*, the uncommon, endemic Del Norte manzanita, with its lightly hairy, 6-8 mm. fruits; *A. viscida* (whiteleaf manzanita) (subsp. *pulchella* and *viscida*), with its sticky, 6-8 mm. fruits; (*The Jepson Manual* on-line). According to Schenck and Gifford (1952:388), the Karuk used *A. canescens*, *A. patula* (greenleaf manzanita) *A. manzanita* (Parry manzanita) and *A. nevadensis* for food. *A. manzanita* grows in the inner and outer North Coast Ranges. *A. patula* grows in the high Cascade Range. Schenck and Gifford (ibid.) describe the processing of Manzanita berries for food as follows:

> The berries are gathered when ripe. The acorn basket (aship) is taken to the bush and the bush is shaken so the berries fall into the basket. They are then spread out in a flat basket (muruk) to dry in the sun and are stored in a storage basket (ashipparakam). The dried berries are sometimes pounded, mixed with salmon eggs, cooked in a basket with hot rock [sic], and eaten.

A drink is made by letting the berries soak in water, straining the water through a basket plate, or allowing the water to percolate through the berries. This is a "good" drink.

See also: oak. For more about poison oak remedies, see also: dandelion, mullein, plantain, ribbed and wide-leaf, soaproot, Solomon seal, walnut, black, wormwood (mugwort), and oatmeal and ocean water in the non-herbal cures section.

Milkweed

Milkweed. Photo by Jennifer Kalt.

KARUK NAME: mitimshaxvuh'íppa ["popping-gum-bush"]

LATIN NAME: *Asclepias eriocarpa*

NATIVE PLANT: Yes

PART USED: The *"milk."*

USE: Used for wart removal and to expel kidney stones: *For kidney stones it takes a while… [T]he gooseberry works a lot faster.* Also used for gum.

PREPARATION: This medicine can only be obtained and used in the spring. Bleed the milk from the cut stems. For wart removal, apply the fresh milk. The milk can't be stored in a jar for more than a few days. Put the milk on the cotton of a Band-Aid, or soak cotton in it, then apply with adhesive tape. *Castor oil is another good thing to get rid of warts. You just keep saturating the wart with castor oil, and in just a few days it'll be gone…*

For kidney stones also use the milk.

For gum, Josephine and her siblings gathered the sap on river bars near the Old Home Place. *We'd go out and cut it, and let it drip in a jar, and save that "milk." Then we'd take it home and put hot water on it, and it would gel up. We'd use it for gum. We'd chew it. My mom used to spill lots of hot boiling water on it. We'd all chew it.*

DOSAGE: For wart removal, apply three to four times a day, and let it dry. Keep applying until the wart disappears. For kidney stones, take about half a teaspoon of the milk two to three times a day for two or three days: *Of course kidney stones are a little rough, where gall stones are smooth and harder. I always go for the gooseberry, because that's safe.*

Only one species of milkweed grows in the local area: *Up on the Old Home, it grew on the river bar. Mom used to tell us, "Don't touch it now." She'd go down with a jar, cut it clear off, and stick it in there, and it'd all run off.*

Schenck and Gifford published the following description of milkweed gum making during a July 1939 field study of Karuk plant use:

When the stem is very fresh, the Karok [sic] break it partway through in many places and catch the milk in a musselshell spoon, a leaf, or some other receptacle. Early morning is the best time for this operation. When enough juice is gathered, it is stirred and heated slightly until it congeals, when it is used as chewing-gum. Putting salmon fat or deer grease on it makes it hold together better in chewing; otherwise it goes to pieces quickly. Both young and old chew the gum, especially at World Renewal gatherings (pikiavish). The fibers are not used for cordage. (1952:388)

See also: gooseberry.

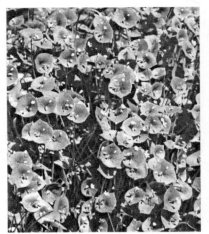

Miner's lettuce.
Photo by Deborah E. McConnell.

Miner's lettuce

LATIN NAME: *Claytonia perfoliata* subsp. *perfoliata*

NATIVE PLANT: Yes

PART USED: Stem, leaves, and flowers.

USE: Laxative and colon cleanser.

PREPARATION: This plant serves as a springtime body cleanser. Eat the leaves fresh. They can be added to salads.

DOSAGE: Eat as much as you can for two days, then follow with six weeks of a blood purifier, such as heal-all.

Miner's lettuce contains the same nutrients as chickweed and is used the same way.

Josephine doesn't recall ever being taught about this plant. As children, she and her siblings would use miner's lettuce to "play dogs," as they called the game. They'd peel the stem, leaving a little "*wire*" or "*cord*" (vein) attached to the round-leafed "*head*" (top) of the plant: *We'd fight one another to see whose head came off first. We'd knock the heads toward each other.* The goal of this contest was to see whose head was the strongest by trying to catch onto another's, then pull it off.

See also: chickweed and psyllium.

Mistletoe

KARUK NAME: anach'úhish (mistletoe, *P. villosum*) ["crow-seed"]

LATIN NAME: *Phoradendron villosum*

NATIVE PLANT: Yes

PART USED: The stem and leaves, although Josephine generally picks off and uses the leaves.

USE: Calming and settling when nervous. Use for convulsions and epilepsy in combination with lady slipper.

PREPARATION: Withheld due to dangerous qualities of the plant.

DOSAGE: Dosage withheld due to dangerous qualities of the plant. *You've got to be careful with the mistletoe. Mistletoe can be poisonous, and it will also abort.*

When Josephine was growing up, people fixed mistletoe tea for individuals who had convulsions and fits, including a young neighbor with epilepsy. *I saw a lot of old people use it for birth control... I never watched how much they made. I never saw them use it much for heart trouble. They always went for the choke-cherry and the dogwood bark.*

P. densum (dense mistletoe), *P. libocedri* (incense cedar mistletoe), and *P. villosum* (oak mistletoe) all grow in the Klamath Ranges Floristic Province.

See also: choke-cherry and dogwood.

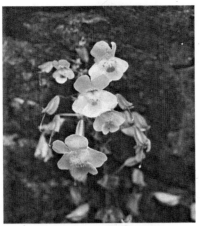

Yellow monkeyflower. Photo by Beverly Ortiz.

Monkeyflower, yellow

KARUK NAME: ikshassahánnihich iiftihan ["one-who-grows-up-in-little-brushy-places"]

LATIN NAME: *Mimulus guttatus*

NATIVE PLANT: Yes

PART USED: Use the entire top of the plant.

USE: Reduces fever.

PREPARATION: Always use fresh. Steep as a tea.

DOSAGE: Take a teaspoon steeped in hot water twice a day, every day, until the fever goes down.

We always used it.

See also: elderberry and Johnny-jump-up.

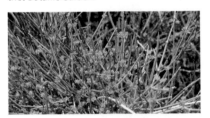

Mormon tea (*Ephedra viridis*). Photo courtesy East Bay Regional Park District Botanic Garden.

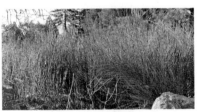

Mormon tea, pollen cones (*Ephedra nevadensis*). Photo courtesy East Bay Regional Park District Botanic Garden.

Mormon tea[36]

aka Indian tea, a common name that Josephine sometimes uses when referring to yerba buena tea

LATIN NAME: *Ephedra* sp. *E. nevadensis* and *E. viridis* grow in the vicinity of Mono Lake, where Josephine gathered this plant.

NATIVE PLANT: Native to desert areas in California.

PART USED: Stem-like leaves.

USE: Blood purifier and diuretic. Used to treat gonorrhea and syphilis.

PREPARATION: Steep a teaspoon in one cup of hot water. Strain out the plant material.

DOSAGE: For blood purifier, take twice a day for six weeks. For diuretic, take once. For gonorrhea, take four times a day until healed.

We used to go around Mono Lake and get it... Clarence Atwell used to give it to Bill Wright, and Bill would bring it to me. (Josephine used to work quite a bit with Bill Wright, an herb doctor from Cortina.)

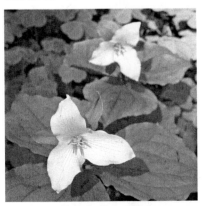

Motherwort. Photo by Beverly Ortiz.

Motherwort (dwarf trillium)

KARUK NAME: annúphiich (trillium, *T. ovatum*)

LATIN NAME: *Trillium ovatum* subsp. *ovatum*

NATIVE PLANT: Yes

PART USED: Bulbs

USE: Labor pains.

PREPARATION: Josephine usually uses the bulb fresh, but you can also dry it. Soak dried bulbs in water prior to use.

DOSAGE: As with Solomon's seal, women in labor should hold a single bulb between their gums and teeth, and suck on it.

See also: Solomon's seal.

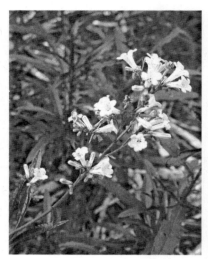

Mountain balm. Photo by Jennifer Kalt.

Mountain balm (yerba santa)

KARUK NAME: pirish'axvâaharas

LATIN NAME: *Eriodictyon californicum*

NATIVE PLANT: Yes

PART USED: Leaves and stem of the new growth (no flower).

USE: Eases flu symptoms. Good for drug babies, asthma and whooping cough. Used with horehound to make a cough syrup. Used with choke-cherry and heal-all to make a cough, asthma, bronchitis, whooping cough, and pneumonia syrup. Firefighters take it to relieve lung congestion caused by smoke. Use with heal-all, Oregon grape root, and yerba buena for cirrhosis of liver, or when the kidneys are giving out.

PREPARATION: Steep as a tea to ease flu symptoms. For details on the preparation and use of syrups with mountain balm, see the section on cough syrups in "Types of Medicinals." Add marijuana to the syrup when used for asthma and whooping cough. For cirrhosis of the liver, or when the kidneys are giving out, steep as a tea.

DOSAGE: For the flu, use an even amount of mountain balm and horehound, together with a handful of marijuana leaves. Adults should take two teaspoons of the syrup whenever they have a coughing fit. For cirrhosis of the liver and kidney disease, steep about half a cup each of the mountain balm, heal-all, Oregon grape root, and yerba buena in a gallon of boiled water. Patients in the last stages of disease can drink it whenever they want.

Josephine distinguishes two types of mountain balm, one she uses, the other she doesn't. Hers are relatively little and short, with a single stem, and grow among sagebrush. The type she doesn't use grows big and bushy, with relatively large leaves.

During the 1999 Meagram Fire, which lasted for about three months and burned some 125,000 acres, Josephine prescribed a syrup of horehound, mountain balm, and marijuana to ease the stuffed-up effect that smoke in the lungs had on fire fighters and cook camp personnel.

When Josephine was growing up, she made plugs of "*tobacco*" from mountain balm leaves: *We'd pick the leaves along the trail. We'd find a nice, smooth rock, and we'd put it on there, then put another heavy rock on top. Leave it there for two or three days, and it would be all smashed together.* After chewing on the plug, Josephine would hurry to get a drink of cold water from a nearby stream or creek, which resulted in a nice, sweet taste.

See also: horehound, heal-all, Oregon grape root, and yerba buena.

Mullein, wild (mule ears)

aka turkey mullein, a common name that Josephine does not use; mule ears is a common name usually applied to *Wyethia* spp., a genus of native sunflowers

LATIN NAME: *Verbascum thapsus*

NATIVE PLANT: No, but locally naturalized: *It's always been around as long as I've been around… It used to grow in the river bars.*

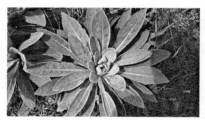

Mullein. Photo by Beverly Ortiz.

PART USED: Leaves. *There's a lot of medicine* [sulphur] *in that flower... I never got into* [using] *the little black seed. I never let it dry.*

USE: The sulphur in mullein is useful for treating sores. Poultice any type of sore. Make a soak or wash for treating ulcerated sores, but not impetigo. Make salve with dandelion and plantain for treating skin diseases (sunburn, eczema, poison oak, and psoriasis), and dry skin, such as on the elbows. Make salve with the same plants for treating boils, ulcerated sores, and skin diseases, like psoriasis, scabies, mange, and ringworm). Make salve with cottonwood and ribbed plantain for treating sores that don't heal.

Make a tea for breathing problems (congested lungs), including asthma, hay fever and bronchitis. Make a tea for hemorrhage of the bowel and lungs, and glandular swelling. Make a tea for bladder and kidney infections. *Sulphur is what they give you when you go to a doctor* [for bladder infections]. [....] *I used to see my mother using it all the time for bladder and kidney problems.*

PREPARATION: For details on the preparation and use of poultices, see the section on poultices in "Types of Medicinals." For ulcerated sores, it's best to soak the affected parts, but a wash may also be used. For the wash, place a strong solution of the tea in a basin. For details on the preparation and use of soaks and washes, see the sections on soaks and washes in "Types of Medicinals."

For the tea, Josephine often harvests two of the big, felty leaves: *We always used to use it fresh. I dry it for winter, but we've had such mild winters now, it grows all winter long.*

DOSAGE: The stronger the wash, the more effective it is. Wash sores three to four times a day. Apply salve periodically until skin has healed.

For tea, Josephine recommends steeping a heaping teaspoon of mullein in one cup of hot water and steeping for one half hour. Using this ratio of herb to water isn't critical, however, although the tea shouldn't be allowed to darken. *It doesn't make any difference, because it isn't going to hurt you.* The tea turns a yellowish green, and can be kept, strained of leaves, for no more than two days. *It'll turn dark if you let it sit too long.* Take one cup of mullein tea in the morning and one in the evening.

Most bladder and kidney infections will clear up in two or three days. *You can take it* [the tea] *several times. We take it for a couple of days, and maybe stop a day or two, and then take it again. Take it for a week or so if you have a lot of bladder infections...*

Although mullein doesn't draw as well as peppernuts, it's useful, as a salve component, for treating ulcerated sores.

When Josephine was growing up, all the old people used salves: *A long time ago in school everybody got impetigo. I don't know whether it was from us playing in the mud, or something else. Of course, that's contagious, and we used to use that* [mullein as a salve] *to try to get rid of it...*

Although Josephine no longer remembers the details, she recalls, as a young child, making salves with her paternal grandmother.

See also: cottonwood, dandelion, and plantain, ribbed. For more about poison oak remedies, see also: dandelion, manzanita, plantain, ribbed and wide-leaf, soaproot, Solomon seal, walnut, black, wormwood (mugwort), and oatmeal and ocean water in the non-herbal cures section.

Mushrooms: tanoak, chanterelle, and commercial

KARUK NAME: xáyviish (*T. magnivelare*)

LATIN NAME: *Tricholoma magnivelare* (synonym *Armillaria ponderosa*)
(tanoak mushroom)
Cantherellus cibarius (chanterelle)
Agaricus bisporus (commercial mushroom)

NATIVE PLANT: Yes, yes, and no respectively.

PART USED: Fruiting body.

USE: Reduction of high blood pressure. Any kind of mushroom will lower blood pressure: *I think that at one of the medical schools, they said it's a sedative medicine.*

PREPARATION: Eat raw, and add to soup and salads. Can, as well.

DOSAGE: Eat four or five a day.

The wholesale destruction of native mushrooms by commercial over-harvesting has become a major concern in Klamath/Trinity River country. If you use native mushrooms, please harvest only a few, taking care not to damage the mycelium in the process, nor to reveal the location.

Mustard, yellow

LATIN NAME: *Brassica rapa* (aka field mustard)

NATIVE PLANT: No, but locally naturalized.

PART USED: Flowers with their little stems.

USE: Relieves congestion of bad chest colds.

PREPARATION: Gather the flowers, including their little stems, and dry. Poultice on at night, akin to a mustard plaster. Wrap flannel over the poulticed flowers. Cover with a damp wash rag, then plastic to keep the poultice moist. The plastic also keeps the dampness away from other clothing and bedding.

Alternatively, make a mustard plaster by mixing about a tablespoon of powdered mustard with half a cup of flour and an egg. Since powdered mustard can burn (blister) the skin, fold the plaster between two layers of flannel, apply, then cover with plastic.

DOSAGE: Unlike powdered mustard, mustard flowers don't burn. The poultice is useful for treating both children and adults, but care must be taken when treating babies.

Apply every night until the congestion breaks.

When Josephine was a child, her family obtained powdered mustard from the Raleigh man. While Josephine uses *Brassica rapa* and *B. nigra* the same way, the former grows relatively close to Josephine's Hoopa Valley home, while the latter grows further away. A field of *Brassica rapa* was plowed up and replaced with grapevines ca. 2008.

Myrrh

LATIN NAME: *Commiphora myrrha* is sold commercially as myrrh.

NATIVE PLANT: No. The plant referred to by this name in herb stores is native to Eastern Africa, especially Somalia.

PART USED: Unknown. Obtained commercially in health food store.

USE: Used with slippery elm for bad breath, sore throat, and tonsillitis. The two plants can also be used separately for sore throats and tonsillitis.

PREPARATION: Steep a "*pinch*" of myrrh and about a quarter of a teaspoonful of powdered slippery elm in about a quarter of a cup of previously-boiled water. Gargle when cooled to a lukewarm temperature.

DOSAGE: Make enough solution to gargle two to three times during a day. Gargle three times a day for sore throat. While it's possible to take too much myrrh, it is safe to use it in a gargle with slippery elm. Do not swallow myrrh. For preparation details, see the section on gargles in "Types of Medicinals."

Myrrh is pronounced "mī-ruh" by Josephine: *You see it growing once in a while. I've seen it growing in Red Bluff. It used to grow where the highway goes through, down in the hollow there, but it wasn't good to get it there, because it's so close to the highway...* This danger results from exhaust pollutants settling on the plants.

Josephine isn't sure when she first learned about myrrh. *It's an antiseptic. You see it in all the mouthwashes, if you look at the ingredients.*

See also: slippery elm.

Nettle

KARUK NAME: akviin (nettle, *U. dioica* subsp. *holosericea*)
neevxâat (coast nettle, *U. dioica* subsp. *gracilis*) ["stinking armpit"]

LATIN NAME: Probably *Urtica dioica* subsp. *gracilis*

NATIVE PLANT: *U. dioica* subsp. *gracilis* (synonym *U. californica*), is native to the United States and Canada, including the North Central coast and Northwestern California, including the Klamath Ranges. *U. dioica* subsp. *holosericea* (synonym *U. holosericea*) is native to Eurasia. It grows in the high Cascade Range.

PART USED: Unknown for blood purifier. Leaves for other purposes.

USE: Blood purifier. Cold and tuberculosis preventative.

PREPARATION: Unknown for blood purifier. For cold preventative, steep ten leaves in a quart of water. To keep the tea strong, don't remove the leaves after making the tea. For tuberculosis preventative, steep two teaspoons of fresh leaves in a cup of water.

DOSAGE: *They* [elders] *say nettle is a good blood purifier, but I've never messed with it, because there's a lot of other stuff we get.* For cold and tuberculosis preventative, drink as much as you want.

Josephine never saw the old people use nettle as a blood purifier. Her mother made a tea for Josephine and her siblings to drink as a tuberculosis preventative.

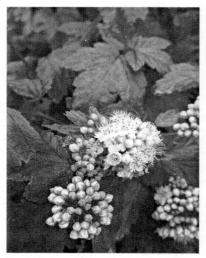

Ninebark. Photo by Jennifer Kalt.

Ninebark

KARUK NAME: tapasxávish ["real-mock-orange"]

LATIN NAME: *Physocarpus capitatus*

NATIVE PLANT: Yes

PART USED: Bark

USE: Stomach or intestinal ulcers, internal cancers (such as in the throat).

PREPARATION: Once home with the bark, dip it in water and shake it off to clean. Steep in hot water to make a tea.

DOSAGE: Use a teaspoon to one cup of hot water: *You've got to take it in small quantities... You've got to take a tablespoonful at a time. Taking any more is going to make you sick.* Take once or twice a day.

Ninebark grows where it's damp. You generally find it where Indians have camped years ago. They brought it in from the coast. The leaf looks similar to a currant.

A Yurok woman from Crescent City area prescribed ninebark to Josephine: *Oh, that's a bitter, nasty thing... She wanted me to take it six weeks, but I couldn't do it... I get goose bumps just thinking about it. There's...nicer tasting things for it now. We've got the wild peach and grindelia.*

See also: grindelia and peach, wild.

Oak

KARUK NAME: xanpúttin (canyon live oak, *Q. chrysolepis*) ["maul-oak-acorn-tree"] axvêep (white oak, *Q. garryana*) ["head-tree"] xánthiip (black Oak, *Q. kelloggii*) [-*ip*: "-tree"]

LATIN NAME: *Quercus* spp. Any species will work for the poultice and eyewash. *Q. chrysolepis* (maul oak, canyon live oak), *Q. garryana* (var. *brewerii* and var. *garryana*) (white oak, aka Oregon oak), *Q. kelloggii* (black oak), *Q. sadleriana* (deer oak), and *Q. vacciniifolia* (huckleberry oak) all grow in the Klamath Ranges (*The Jepson Manual* on-line).

NATIVE PLANT: Yes

PART USED: Acorns and bark.

USE: Poultice for burns. Eyewash for eye infections and cataracts.

PREPARATION: For treating burns, use unleached acorn flour: *With the ones that come here with burns, I use acorn flour. I put boiling water on the flour, make a paste, put it on thick, bandage it, and tell them to leave it there for two days. When you take it off, it's almost healed.* The boiling water sterilizes the paste. The tannins in the flour heal the burn.

Alternatively, for treating burns, burn pieces of oak in the heater stove and save the ashes. Mix some ashes with just enough water to make a paste in your hand. Apply the paste, then poultice. Wrap the paste with flannel or other soft, cotton cloth, then cover with Saran plastic wrap to retain the moisture. Keep the affected part still. For details on the preparation and use of poultices and pastes, see the section on poultices and pastes in "Types of Medicinals."

For treating eye infections and cataracts, retain the first batch of acorn-leaching water. Put a flat basket with a porous cloth over a glass (never metal)

Black oak. Photo courtesy East Bay Regional Park District Botanic Garden.

bowl. Put acorn flour atop the cloth. Drip lukewarm water through the acorn, catching the first water in the bowl. For details on the preparation of acorn leaching water, see the acorn subsection in the nuts section of "Native Plant Foods."

DOSAGE: Apply paste thickly to burns. After two days, upon removal of the poultice, there should be no evidence of peeling or blistering. For bad burns, it can take three days.

For eye infections and cataracts, mix one tablespoon of tannin water and two tablespoons of boiled water. Wash eyes once or twice a day. Eye infections should clear up in two days. To keep cataracts off, wash eyes for three to four days, then quit. Do this every time you "*soak*" (leach) acorns.

The tannin in oaks is useful for treating severe burns: *You put the tannin on when you get burned, and that draws out the hurt. If you bandage the ashes on, and keep it there, it won't blister.* Josephine used acorn as an eyewash in the 1980s and successfully cleared up specks in her own eyes.

See also: oak, white and tanoak. For an alternative burn remedy, see manzanita.

Oak, white

aka Oregon oak, a common name that Josephine does not use

KARUK NAME: axvêep ["head-tree"]

LATIN NAME: *Quercus garryana*

NATIVE PLANT: Yes

PART USED: Acorns, wood, and bark.

USE: Poultice for burns. Eyewash for eye infections and cataracts. Tea for gallstones, and kidney stones, and the reduction of fevers.

PREPARATION: For treating burns, use unleached flour or burn pieces of oak in the heater stove and save the ashes. For treating eye infections and cataracts, retain the first batch of acorn-leaching water. For details about treating burns, eye infections, and cataracts, *see* Oak.

For gallstones, kidney stones, and the reduction of fevers, make a tea from the inner bark: *We mostly take the new growth that you can peel off. After the bark gets thick it's hard to make anything out of it… You can chop the outer bark off and use the inner bark.*

DOSAGE: For burns, eye infections, and cataracts, see "Oak." Unknown for gallstones, kidney stones, and reduction of fevers.

As a child, Josephine saw her maternal Grandma Bennett use the inner bark, but didn't notice how much was taken. Both grandmothers used herbs, as did others of their generation, because doctors weren't available.

White oak. Photo courtesy East Bay Regional Park District Botanic Garden.

White oak, detail. Photo courtesy East Bay Regional Park District Botanic Garden.

Onion, wild

KARUK NAME: xannáachyuh (*A. acuminatum*) ["a-little-long-downriverward"]

pufichxannáchyuh (wild onion, *A. bolanderi*) ["Deer-a-little-long-downriver"]

LATIN NAME: *Allium acuminatum*

NATIVE PLANT: Yes

PART USED: Bulb

USE: Food

PREPARATION: Dig while in bloom. Eat raw. Cook in stews, or make into a chowder, akin to potato soup, substituting wild onions for commercial ones.

DOSAGE: N/A

Josephine and her siblings dug wild onions as children. She digs them with a T-shaped tool that curved on the digging end. For a fuller description of this tool, see Indian potato.

The local wild onion has a cluster of white flowers on top of the stalk, giving it the appearance of an Indian potato. Josephine has gathered wild onions wherever she could, including near Cloverdale, California, and Tahlequah, Oklahoma. She fondly recalls the latter experience, when a woman whose home was surrounded by a pasture gathered some and made them into soup: *It was the best tasting thing.*

Of the fourteen species of wild onion that grow in the Klamath Ranges Floristic Province, two are native to Europe (*A. paniculatum* var. *paniculatum* and *A. vineale*), four are uncommon (*A. cratericola, A. membranaceum, A. siskiyouense,* and *A. unifolium*), and four others lack white blossoms, or grow in the wrong soil substrate (*A. bolanderi, A. campanulatum, A. falcifolium, A. hoffmanii,* and *A. validum*). Of the remaining two, *A. acuminatum*, with its ten to forty white to rose-purple blossoms, grows in hills and plains, whereas *A. amplectens*, with its ten to fifty white to pink flowers, is limited to clay soils, including serpentine (*The Jepson Manual* on-line). *A. acuminatum* and *A. bolanderi* were identified as having been eaten by the Karuk during a July 1939 field study (Schenck and Gifford 1952:380).

Oregon grape

KARUK NAME: ihyivkâanvar / thukinpírish ["shouting-down-over-instrument" / "bile-plant"]

LATIN NAME: *Berberis nervosa*

NATIVE PLANT: Yes

PART USED: Root

USE: *Any herb that turns yellow when you make a tea is good for the liver. It cleanses the liver. Like the Oregon grape root. We take that for a blood purifier.* Also take for pancreatitis, liver and kidney problems. Use with mountain balm leaves, heal-all leaves, grape root, and yerba buena leaves for cirrhosis of the liver or when the kidneys are giving out.

PREPARATION: Gather the root, scrub it off with a wire brush, chop it up, and dry it. Store it in a jar: *Now you can get it chopped up finely in a health food store.*

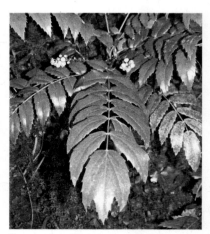

Oregon grape. Photo by Jennifer Kalt.

If you say you want fresh, they'll get it for you... I think they peel it somehow. To make a blood purifier, steep a week's dosage as a tea in a gallon jar. Store the jar in the refrigerator.

DOSAGE: For a blood purifier, make in the standard dosage of a teaspoon to one cup of hot water. This is the equivalent of about eight pencil-sized or smaller roots to a quart of hot water. Leave the herb in the water so it strengthens during storage. Take one cup in the morning and one in the evening for six weeks in the fall and spring: *In the fall, maybe October or November, you start using the grape to cleanse your system. It keeps you from getting colds and flu during the winter months.*

For pancreatitis, take one cup a day for one month to six weeks to prevent further attacks.

For cirrhosis of the liver and kidney disease, use about one tablespoon each of the mountain balm, heal-all, and yerba buena mixture to a quart of water, or about half a cup each to a gallon of water. Sip two cups' worth throughout the day. Take for two weeks, then stop. Wait ten days, then resume as needed. Patients in the last stages of disease can drink it whenever they want.

There are two species of Oregon grape: a domestic one that grows about four feet high, and the one Josephine uses, which grows along the ground, then comes up in clumps.

Josephine learned about Oregon grape through the Chinese herbalist whose sons she befriended.

See also: dock, yellow, goldenseal, mountain balm, heal-all, and yerba buena.

Parsley

LATIN NAME: *Petroselinum crispum*

NATIVE PLANT: No, but cultivated locally

PART USED: Stem and leaves.

USE: Diuretic and breath freshener. High in vitamin B and potassium; contains a substance in which tumorous cells cannot multiply.

PREPARATION: Eat raw for diuretic. After eating garlic, chew on parsley to freshen breath.

DOSAGE: Eat two pieces (*that's plenty*) for several days.

I don't know how we came by it as a medicine. We always had parsley growing up high [off the ground in buckets or wooden boxes], *so the dogs didn't pee in it. We'd use it in our salads. My mom always used to chop it up fine and put it in the potato salad, and they always put it in the stews. They put it on your plate all the time in restaurants. They* [Josephine's older relatives] *always told us it helps your heart. We used to throw it off to the side, and they'd eat it.*

Until she was eight or nine years old, Josephine had only boys to play with—five brothers and uncles. *We ate garlic on the sly* [laughs]. *We did it just to see who could eat the most...* To eliminate the resultant bad breath, she needed only to chew parsley.

Passion Flower

LATIN NAME: *Passiflora* spp.

NATIVE PLANT: No, but several species cultivated in nurseries locally.

PART USED: Unknown

USE: A sedative used for treating individuals who are "keyed up" or evidence "hysteria," including from menopause. Symptoms include headache, neuralgia, and high blood pressure.

PREPARATION: Unknown

DOSAGE: Unknown

Passion flower, a vine native to Hawaii, has lovely chartreuse pink or red flowers, and Josephine has a small vine of it growing in a pot in her home. She recalls learning about its medicinal value while living in southern California in the early 1960s: *They always said it was good for people that get hysteria. They give it to calm them down. It's just something that they told me, and it stuck with me.* Josephine doesn't prescribe this plant.

Peach, domestic

LATIN NAME: *Prunus persica*

NATIVE PLANT: No, but cultivated locally.

PART USED: Leaves

USE: Relaxer. Eases morning sickness (settles the stomach). Arrests symptoms if you notice a flu coming on.

PREPARATION: Use fresh or dried.

DOSE: Steep two leaves in one cup of hot water. For morning sickness, drink <u>only</u> two doses a day.

For relaxing, half a cup is enough. To ward off flu or colds, Josephine adds a half teaspoon of chamomile. To prevent flu, two cups is enough.

Peach leaf tea should be taken judiciously, since it lowers the blood pressure. Although the tea has a nice flavor, like Labrador tea, it will build up a toxic poison if allowed to sit, and can cause stroke—so make only one dose at a time.

Momma used to make [peach] *tea every time she got pregnant... Eleven times! Eleven times she was pregnant. And I always saw her fixing up these leaves...*

Peach, wild (oso berry)

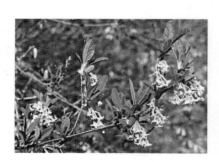
Wild peach. Photo by Beverly Ortiz

LATIN NAME: *Oemleria cerasiformis*

NATIVE PLANT: Yes

PART USED: Stem. Don't use the leaves, flowers or berries, as they're poisonous.

USE: Cancer treatment, taken after drinking a tea made from grindelia tops.

PREPARATION: Break up the little stems. Steep as a tea.

DOSAGE: If consumed in large quantities, wild peach can be poisonous. Put about four one-inch pieces of stem in one cup of hot water. Drink about half a cup of grindelia, wait half an hour, then drink half a cup of the wild peach. The grindelia settles the stomach so the wild peach will stay down. Take both twice a day for about three weeks: *All of the sudden you'll get really sick, and you'll vomit what will look like a bunch of hair. This is fevers of the cancer coming out. A lot of patients will only take it just so long, then quit. They get scared when they get sick. But you take it three weeks, then you stop for a week or two, then you take it again.*

You can make a quart of wild peach stem tea at a time, but Josephine prefers to make it fresh each time.

Flora Jones (Wintun) called this plant wild peach. Josephine has known about it all her life. Wild peach contains arsenic, which Josephine finds to be beneficial for HIV/AIDS patients.

See also: grindelia.

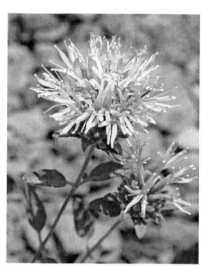

Pennyroyal. Photo by Jennifer Kalt.

Pennyroyal (coyote mint)

Josephine uses these names interchangeably. She also uses a German species of pennyroyal.

KARUK NAME: thámkaat ["meadow-mugwort"]

LATIN NAME: *Monardella odoratissima*

NATIVE PLANT: Yes

PART USED: The above-ground parts of the plant (leaves, stem, and flowers).

USE: Take when you feel the headache and fever symptoms of a cold coming on, or to treat a cold or fever. Also take for convulsions and "female troubles" (menstrual cramps and a heavy flow).

PREPARATION: Pick pennyroyal before it flowers. Although pennyroyal can be used fresh or dried, Josephine dries hers for practical reasons: *By the time you pick it and get it home, it's nearly dry anyway.* Pennyroyal tea can sit, so Josephine makes it by the quart and stores it in the refrigerator.

DOSAGE: Don't take if you're pregnant, as this plant can cause abortions. Use a teaspoon of the herb to one cup of hot water. To knock out the symptoms of a cold, drink three cupfuls in close succession. For colds and fevers, drink pennyroyal hot several times a day.

For cramps take the tea two to three times a day, once in the morning and again in the evening, or an additional cup at midday. *You can drink pennyroyal all the time, but you don't take it if you're pregnant, because it'll abort. That's probably why my kids are twenty years apart,* Josephine quipped with a laugh.

There are two types of pennyroyal, a native one that grows out of bedrock cliff-faces along the highway, and appears somewhat bushy, with flowers growing in clusters, and a short, non-native, German species with a smaller flower. Although the native species is gathered before it flowers, the German species, which grows at higher elevations near Greenville, has already flowered by the time Josephine can access it, after the snow melts. *Around here it grows in big bunches. The German one comes out with one shoot and a little purple flower... We've used both of them.*

Josephine used to drink coyote mint tea once in a while for pleasure. She saw it used for convulsions due to aneurysm, stroke and epilepsy in children, although, when treating convulsions herself, she uses mistletoe and white lady slipper. She attributes convulsions to brain damage caused by aneurysm, stroke, and, at times, from more mundane causes: *A lot of people can feel convulsions coming on before they get them. Some people who get them just drop. I could feel them coming on if I got too tired doing something.*

Peppermint

LATIN NAME: *Mentha piperita*

NATIVE PLANT: No, but planted in gardens locally.

PART USED: Tops of the plants. Root not used.

USE: Gas pain (indigestion). Add to goldenseal, blood root and some other liquid herbal medicines for taste. If capsules are used, peppermint is unnecessary for taste.

PREPARATION: Let the root dry to reduce the juice, but don't let it become so dry it becomes hard. Next, pound it up, then store it.

DOSAGE: Steep one teaspoon of the pounded root in one cup of hot water for indigestion. When adding peppermint to goldenseal or blood root, use only a little bit, just enough to taste good to you. As with other teas, don't pour boiling water over the herb, just steep to make the tea.

While growing up, Josephine drank peppermint tea for pure enjoyment.

See also: ginger, goldenseal, and blood root.

Peppernut (bay, bay laurel)

aka myrtlewood in Oregon

KARUK NAME: pahiip ["bay-nut-tree"]

LATIN NAME: *Umbellularia californica*

NATIVE PLANT: Yes

PART USED: Leaves and nutmeat.

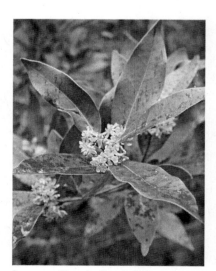

Peppernut. Photo by Beverly Ortiz.

USE: Aromatic steam from heated leaves for colds and sinus infections. New growth (young, light green leaves on tips of branches) for toothache. Leaves for shingles. Mashed, fresh nutmeats preferred to other herbs by Josephine for drawing out boils and blood poisoning caused by stepping on nails, snake bites, spider bites, fish bone injuries, and any type of sores, such as diabetic sores, bedsores, and impetigo. It's also used for spider bites: *The meat in that little peppernut is the best medicine there is for boils or blood poisoning, snake bites... It'll draw it right out... I've cured a lot of diabetic sores, people that have it on their feet... It's great for impetigo.* Peppernut meat can be applied to the swelling of infections, although Josephine prefers wormwood for this purpose. Nutmeats roasted and eaten to prevent allergies in the spring, colds and flu in the fall, and to relieve colitis and ulcers. Oil used for earaches.

PREPARATION: For information about gathering, cleaning, drying and roasting peppernuts, see the subsection on peppernuts in the nuts section of "Native Plant Foods." *If we're catching a cold or have sinus problems, I put* [boiling water in] *a* [coffee] *can on the stove, then put leaves in, and let the aroma go through the house.* Alternatively, for sinuses, boil water in a pot, then add the leaves. Put a towel over your head and breathe the steam.

To relieve the pain of a toothache, rub the young, new growth leaves back and forth in your hands to release the oils, then lay these oily leaves around your tooth. For shingles, Josephine removes the largest leaves she can from the branches, then dips or soaks them in a pan of hot water to release the oils. She then creates a poultice of the leaves with a piece of flannel or gauze. Although the poultice stings when applied, it dries up the blisters and prevents others from reccurring. Constantly replace the leaves, keeping them warm. Shingles generally clear up in two to three days. Alternately, make a very strong solution of the leaves in a pan of hot water, then dip a washrag into it. Josephine's uncle made just such a wash, storing it in a gallon jar, with the leaves inside. He'd reheat it as needed. For preparation details, see the section on soaks in "Types of Medicinals."

For boils, blood poisoning and sores, poultice a peppernut plaster on the wound. Both fresh and older stored nuts can be used. Chop the raw nut up finely in a chopper and add just enough olive oil to make the plaster. Josephine used to crush the raw nuts in a mortar; now she uses a mini food mill. Use a round bandage to hold the plaster in place on the wound. Josephine poultices diabetic sores, which generally occur on the toes and heel, with plastic gloves. *You feel it within twenty minutes. It draws so hard, sometimes you can hardly stand it.* The plaster can get hard, but when you heat it, it softens again due to its oil content.

For flu and cold preventative, and for treating colitis and ulcers, eat the roasted nuts. See the subsection on peppernuts in the nuts section of "Native Plant Foods" for roasting instructions.

About preparing peppernuts for treating ear aches, Josephine had this to say: *We used to crack peppernuts, mash them up, and put them in a* [teacup] *saucer on the back of our heating stove. The oils will drip out. You just mash it up a little bit so the oil will leak out faster. We saved that oil. If you had a bad ear ache or infection inside the ear, you'd just drop that oil in.*

DOSAGE: *The smell keeps your sinuses open, but you can't get too close, because it'll burn up in your head* [laughs].

Each poultice generally remains in place about five or six hours.

Blood poisoning is sometimes caused by redwood[37] slivers and fish bones. It causes streaks to form along blood veins. When a streak appears, apply a poultice and, within two hours, it should recede. Apply a second poultice to insure the infection has been completely eliminated.

Taking four to five roasted peppernuts a day should be enough to keep one's system immune to flu and colds, although Josephine eats them for enjoyment and doesn't keep track. Eat four to five nuts a day for ulcers and colitis.

Josephine, who refers to the entire plant as a peppernut, learned its uses as a child: *The old timers always used it when we were kids.*

Once, I asked Josephine if her people used this plant for shingles and sores when she was growing up: *They always had it. In summer our Indian myths tell us about the peppernut being the Indian doctor.* Josephine's response alludes to the brush dance, a healing ceremony held in the summertime for a sick child. *The little peppernut would come to the healing dance and roll around in front of the people attending. She'd roll back and forth to let them know she had healing powers.* Josephine's Grandma Grant used to tell stories throughout the year to keep the children in the house and entertained.

As children, Josephine and her siblings roasted the nuts at home. Josephine learned to treat shingles from her uncle, who lived with the family when he was young. Although mullein can be substituted for peppernuts in poultices, it doesn't draw as well, and thus doesn't work as quickly.

A long time ago they used to use the oil from an eel for ear infections: The oil is just fat. You can cook the eel and get all kinds of grease out of it. And then we always had goose grease. We'd kill a goose and render the oil out of it, and save it for when the babies get a bad cold in wintertime. You just saturate them with goose grease… They'd put it on our backs and on our chests.

Josephine attributes the relatively high incidence of colitis in the Klamath and Trinity River areas to a diet rich in jerked and dried salmon.

See also: heal-all, mullein, tobacco, and willow, gray.

Pine

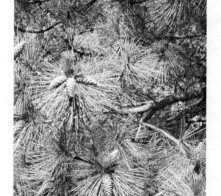

Ponderosa pine. Photo by Jennifer Kalt.

KARUK NAME: ishvakíppish (knobcone pine, *P. attentuata*) ["just-a-little-chin"] ishvírip (Jeffrey pine, *P. jeffreyi*) [(?) + *-ip*, "tree"] ússip (sugar pine, *P. lambertiana*) ishvírip (ponderosa pine, *P. ponderosa*) [(?) + *-ip*, "tree"] axyússip (gray pine, *P. sabiniana*) ["sugar-pine-cone(/-nut)-tree"]

LATIN NAME: *Pinus* spp. Any species will work, although Josephine is most familiar with *P. jeffreyi*, *P. lambertiana*, and *P. ponderosa*.

NATIVE PLANT: Yes

PART USED: Pitch

USE: Stops cuts from bleeding. The turpentine in the pitch kills any infection.

PREPARATION: Cut a "V" in the bark of a pine and collect the pitch. Place soft or juicy pitch on the cut.

DOSAGE: Apply immediately.

When Josephine and her siblings were children, and got cuts, turpentine, which kills infection, was poured on the wound. Josephine remembers that it stung.

P. albicaulis (whitebark pine), *P. attenuata* (knobcone pine), *P. balfouriana* (subsp. boufouriana) (foxtail pine), *P. contorta* (subsp. murrayana) (lodgepole pine), *P. jeffreyi* (Jeffrey pine, *P. lambertiana* (sugar pine), *P. monticola* (western white pine), *P. ponderosa* (ponderosa pine), and *P. sabiniana* (gray pine, foothill pine) grow in the Klamath Ranges (*The Jepson Manual* on-line).

Josephine uses gray pine roots in her basketry.

Pineapple plant (chamomile)

LATIN NAME: Unknown. Possibly *Chamomilla recutita* or *Amthemis arvensis*. The two species of pineapple plant that Josephine uses cannot be *C. occidentalis* or *C. suaveolens*, which is widely known as common pineapple weed, because the species that Josephine uses has "*little, white petals*" (ray flowers), while the latter two species solely have disk flowers. Josephine describes one of the species she uses as growing a foot or more tall, while the other grows close to the ground, maybe six inches high.

NATIVE PLANT: Yes.

PART USED: Flowers

USE: Calms the nerves so you can sleep. Used to stop smoking and drinking, and to withdraw from drugs. Also relieves muscle pain and toothache. Used as a childhood drink.

PREPARATION: Steep as a tea for all uses, except toothache and childhood drink. You can strain out the flowers and keep the tea for a day or so. The flowers may be used dried and fresh. When dried, they lose potency, so use a little more. Store the dried flowers in glass jars to help retain their potency.

For childhood drink, steep top of plant in cold tap water throughout the day or overnight; use lukewarm water to "*hurry it up.*" Strain out the plant parts and add a little sugar to taste.

DOSAGE: Make the tea in the standard ratio of a teaspoon to one cup. Josephine recommends taking one cup in the morning and one in the evening, although chamomile, which isn't dangerous, can be taken in any amount desired. For toothache, chew the flowers fresh, never dried. When young, Josephine and her siblings soaked the flowers in cold water to create a drink that Josephine recalls "*really liking*": *In those days we had to look for good things to drink, as we didn't have anything.*

Chamomile is found in barnyards and open fields.

The need for chamomile to assist with drug withdrawal is an historic phenomenon. Spanish Fly, a crystal imported from Mexico, was one of the earliest drugs to enter the local area.

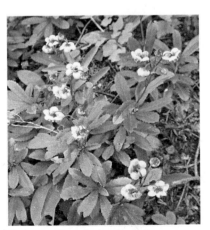

Pipsissewa. Photo by Jennifer Kalt.

Pipsissewa [pip-sō-ē-nuh] (princess pine)

aka prince's pine, a common name that Josephine does not use

KARUK NAME: xunyêepshurukhitihan ["one-who-is-under-tanoak-trees"]

LATIN NAME: *Chimaphila umbellata*

NATIVE PLANT: Yes

PART USED: Leaves and stem.

USE: Bladder problems that result from bad kidneys.

PREPARATION: Steep as a tea.

DOSAGE: Use the standard teaspoon to one cup of hot water, or, if you wish, make the tea a little stronger. Take half a cup four times a day until bladder problems are gone.

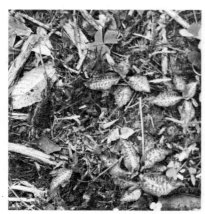

Rattlesnake plantain. Photo by Beverly Ortiz.

Plantain, rattlesnake

KARUK NAME: achnat'apvuytiiv ["dusky-footed-woodrat-tail-cars"]

LATIN NAME: *Goodyera oblongifolia*

NATIVE PLANT: Yes

PART USED: Leaves

USE: Fertility

PREPARATION: Steep one teaspoon of the leaves in one cup of water.

DOSAGE: Take twice a day, once in the morning and evening, for one week after your menstrual cycle ends.

Josephine used to gather rattlesnake plantain as a child at the request of the woman from whom she first learned about herbs.

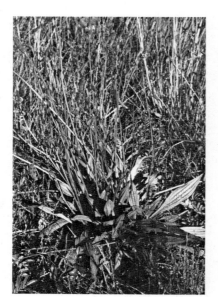

Ribbed plantain. Photo by Beverly Ortiz

Plantain, ribbed (narrow), and wide-leaf plantain

LATIN NAME: *Plantago lanceolata* (ribbed plantain)
Plantago major (wide-leaf plantain)

NATIVE PLANT: No, but locally naturalized.

PART USED: Leaves for bleeding, open sores and skin ulcers. Root for enema or piles; discard the tops or flower.

USE: Enemas used for hemorrhoids. Root for piles. Dried, powdered leaves used to stop bleeding. Fresh leaves applied for wind chap. Leaves poulticed on open sores and skin ulcers. Although dry leaves can be poulticed, it's better to use fresh. Wash for skin diseases, like psoriasis, and rashes (heat and allergic): *Both plantains are good for that* [psoriasis]. *Add a little bit of lanolin... Olive oil is good for psoriasis, too.*

A salve can be made made with dandelion and mullein for skin diseases (sunburn, eczema, poison oak, and psoriasis), and dry skin, such as on the elbows. Salve made with the same plants for skin sores (impetigo, infected sores, and ulcerated sores). Salve made with coltsfoot, wormwood, and garden violet (if pain) for boils, ulcerated sores, and skin diseases, like psoriasis, scabies, mange and ringworm). Salve made with cottonwood for sores that don't heal. Salve made with white clover and dandelion for boils, sores that don't heal, and skin diseases.

PREPARATION: For enemas or piles, dig up the entire plant. Retain the root and leaves, but discard the tops or flower: *I'd go out and dig it and dry it, and put it in pint jars, and use it for an enema. You made it warm, not cold. They always kept it kind of warm.*

Place dry, powdered mullein leaf in open wounds to stop the bleeding. In the past a mortar and pestle was used to powder the leaves. *Everything goes through a coffee grinder now* [laughs]. *Or the grist mill.*

When we kids were little, we used to get that old wind chap from the cold weather. While walking, our hands were always getting wet, and they'd get chapped, and we'd just get the leaves and rub it on.

For preparation details of soaks, washes, poultices, and salves, *see* the sections of washes, poultices, and salves, in "Types of Medicinals."

DOSAGE: For enemas, piles, and soaks, make a strong tea: *My mom had bad hemorrhoids after having a baby. I always used to see her making it strong.*

For enemas or piles, use daily. Soak periodically until healed. Apply washes two to three times per day. Reapply poultices two times per day. Apply salves periodically until healed.

Although plantains aren't native, Josephine remembers her grandmother preparing the powder and the washes for her father: *He worked in cement a lot. Something out of that cement went through him. He'd get carbuncles all the time... I remember we used a lot of Epsom salts for him too, you know, to draw stuff out of it.*

A long time ago in school everybody got impetigo. Of course, that's contagious. Although Josephine no longer remembers the details, she recalls, as a young child, making salves with her paternal grandmother.

See also: clover, white, coltsfoot, cottonwood, dandelion, Johnny-jump-up, mullein, and wormwood. For alternative poison oak remedies, *see also:* dandelion, manzanita, mullein, soaproot, Solomon seal, walnut, black, wormwood (mugwort), and oatmeal and ocean water in the non-herbal cures section.

Pleurisy root

LATIN NAME: Unknown

NATIVE PLANT: Unknown

PART USED: Root

USE: Reduces fevers.

PREPARATION: Peel the bark off the white-colored root, then chop it up in a chopper. Steep as a tea.

DOSAGE: Use the standard teaspoon to one cup of hot water. Drink a maximum of two cups a day until the fever is gone.

"*The old ones*" taught Josephine about pleurisy root. *Asclepias tuberosa* is sold commercially as pleurisy root, but the species Josephine uses is not a milkweed, but rather "*milkweed like.*"

Plum, Klamath

LATIN NAME: *Prunus subcordata*

NATIVE PLANT: Yes

PART USED: Fruit

USE: Food

PREPARATION: Prepare as jelly and jam. For preparation details, *see* the subsection on jams and jellies, in the cooking with fruit section of "Native Plant Foods."

DOSAGE: N/A

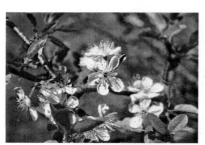

Klamath plum, detail. Photo courtesy East Bay Regional Park District Botanic Garden.

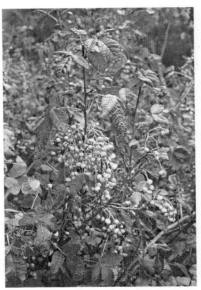

Poison oak. Photo by Jennifer Kalt.

Poison oak

KARUK NAME: kusvêep [kus- (bitter?)] = ["mountain mahogany"]

LATIN NAME: *Toxicodendrom diversilobum* (synonym *Rhus diversiloba*)

NATIVE PLANT: Yes

PART USED: Leaves, stem, juice.

USE: To immune oneself to the rash, and for tattooing.

PREPARATION: Caution: Do not experiment with this plant. Eating poison oak may give a person an intestinal rash or cause death.

To become immune to poisoning, gather and eat two small leaflets in the spring, when they're small and tender. Alternatively, and more rarely for immunity, gather an inch of the stem in the spring, and eat it. For tattoos, scratch the skin and put in juice.

DOSAGE: Withheld due to potential dangers if misused.

As children, Josephine and her siblings ate poison oak "*just to be doing it*," and to show off. Josephine has never gotten the rash. In her experience, if one gets a bad poison oak rash, after future exposure, the skin will only develop itchy spots.

In addition to eating poison oak, Josephine experimented with tattooing her skin with the juice: *We used to take it and scratch our skin and put the juice in it to tattoo, because* [the skin] *turns black. We used to almost get murdered for doing that... We scratched our skin with a needle, then put the juice in it. I don't know whether I put my boyfriend's initials in it, or whether it was mine or something else* [laughs]. Josephine's skin swelled for two or three days after she tattooed her hand. Later, she had the tattoo removed by a doctor.

Josephine doesn't remember how much poison oak she ate, nor does she think she was encouraged to do so: *We had it all over the ranch, so we had to get in it. And when we cut wood, we had to get in it. I think most of the Indians did it to immune themselves. I don't know if we just did it, or our uncles told us to, or what.* Ocean water is Josephine's preferred treatment for poison oak rash: *If you've got poison oak bad, just go swim in the ocean.*

For a Rumsien Ohlone account about eating poison oak, *see* Ortiz (2002).

See also Solomon seal for more on poison oak.

Psyllium

LATIN NAME: *Plantago psyllium*

NATIVE PLANT: No

PART USED: Leaves and stem.

USE: Excellent colon cleanser. Creates bulk. Take with laxative herb. Anti-intoxication.

PREPARATION: Use fresh or dried.

DOSAGE: Eat fresh. Put the dried plant into water to soften it up, then eat it once a day for two days: *I've seen them eat quite a bit, but due to the taste, maybe you can eat a couple of tablespoonfuls.*

Josephine thinks she learned about this herb, which doesn't grow in the local area, from a doctor up by Umatilla: *That's not in our area either. They used to send it to me* [dried], *and we'd go up north and dig it out of Pendleton... They'd use that like we'd use the chickweed and miner's lettuce to cleanse our system.*

See also: chickweed and miner's lettuce.

Purslane

aka pulsane, a common name that Josephine does not use

LATIN NAME: *Portulaca oleracea*

NATIVE PLANT: No, but locally naturalized.

PART USED: Entire plant, except the root, which is small.

USE: For skin rashes, wounds, mouth ulcers (sores), canker sores, gum boils, and as a diuretic. Also for food.

PREPARATION: Purslane may only be used seasonally: *If you try to dry it, you can't. As soon as* [the plants] *get moist, it'll go right back to that watery stage. So you can only use it while it's out... It grows out here in the back garden. It doesn't come up until after you plow, and your garden dies down in about the fall, when it gets a lot of rain. It comes up whenever we have sprinklers going out there. It goes dormant if the rains don't come.*

When she was growing up, Josephine recalls mashing purslane and applying it to skin spots: *When we went swimming in the summertime, we'd get all blotchy. You know, dry spots, and white spots, from being out in the sun. And we used to get it, mash it up, and put it all over.*

For skin rashes and wounds, poultice the crushed, watery stems and leaves. For details on the preparation and use of poultices, see the section on poultices in "Types of Medicinals." Chew the entire above-ground, raw plant—stems, leaves, and flowers—for sores of any type in the mouth.

For a diuretic, boil, then eat purslane. As Josephine quipped: *You can get skinny on it.* About her efforts to stay slim as a teenager, Josephine had this to say: *We've tried it. We've tried everything* [laughs].

For food, purslane can be eaten fresh, added to salads, or boiled like spinach: *We'd eat a lot of it summertime out here, because it grows in the* [Hoopa] *Valley. We used to eat it at home all the time* [when we were growing up]. *We would pick it when it comes up, and eat it as a green.* Put it in salad. When boiled, add vinegar to taste.

DOSAGE: For sores in the mouth of any type, including gum boils, chew the raw plant--stems, leaves, and flowers..

Josephine does not know how many applications of mashed purslane it would take to clear up spots: *We never paid any attention. We just put it on whenever we came to a plant. But it cleared it up. We used to grab it, and squeeze it, because a lot of water comes out, and we'd just rub it on.*

For a diuretic, eat purslane once, akin to taking a water pill. For food, eat as much as desired.

About the extent and appearance of purslane, Josephine shared the following: *In the late summer it grows in gardens. It's a really watery plant, and the stems are kind of red... It has little, yellow flowers on it.* At the Old Home Place, purslane grew along the Salmon River, not far from the family home, and in the family garden: *In the summertime, it stayed damp in the sand close to the river. It grew just nice and juicy... There was water running down to the field, so it always grew in the garden.* A long time ago, purslane was used fresh for scurvy. In addition to boiling purslane like spinach, Josephine's mother also used it as medicine. Although Josephine does not recall eating very much of this plant as a child, she vividly remembers using it to heal a gash, some six inches long, on her arm, caused during a childhood fall while carrying a *"big, white pitcher,"* which shattered into pieces. Someone headed out to the garden to get purslane, while Josephine's brother was sent to the barn to get cobwebs. Purslane juice was applied to the wound, then the cobwebs packed inside it to stop the bleeding.

Reindeer moss (old man's beard)

LATIN NAME: Probably *Usnea* spp., which grows in trees. The species are difficult to identify, even for lichenologists. Some people use the common name reindeer moss for a more coastal, ground-dwelling plant, which is unrelated to lichens in the genus *Usnea*.

NATIVE PLANT: Yes

PART USED: Whole plant.

USE: Sour or upset stomach, flu, sore and strep throats, mouth sores.

PREPARATION: Gather from white oak. *We just chew it up and swallow* [the juice], *because deer eat it... It doesn't have much taste to it...*

DOSAGE: Chew a mouthful. *It isn't going to hurt you, but it will stop a sore throat.*

Josephine recalls chewing this plant and swallowing the juice when she felt a flu or cold coming on. She describes its appearance as "long, white whisker things hanging off" the oak.

The basketry lichen (*Letharia vulpia*), used to dye porcupine quills, is gathered off high elevation fir.

Rose hips

KARUK NAME: achnatsinvánnahich (cluster rose, *R. pisocarpa*) ["little-big-lost-thorn"]

achnatsinvannahichkaam (ground rose, *R. spithamea*) ["little-lost-thorn"]

LATIN NAME: *Rosa* spp. All native species seem to work equally well. *R. californica* (California rose), *R. canina* (dog rose), *R. eglanteria* (sweet-briar), *R. gymnocarpa* (wood rose), *R. nutkana* var. *nutkana* (Nootka rose), *R. pisocarpa* (cluster rose), and *R. spithamea* (ground rose) all grow in the Klamath Ranges (*The Jepson Manual* on-line).

NATIVE PLANT: Yes

PART USED: Fruits (hips) when they turn orange.

USE: Contains natural Vitamin C. When catching a cold, or for diabetes, take as tea. Apply to bee stings, mosquito bites, and other insect bites.

PREPARATION: Use fresh or dried for tea. To dry, first cut the hip in half or chop it up. Use fresh for stings and bites. Cut the fresh hip in half, then rub the juice on the affected area.

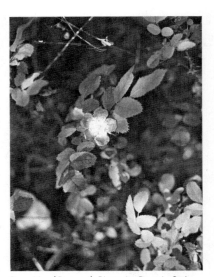

Rose hips (*Rosa* sp.). Photo by Beverly Ortiz.

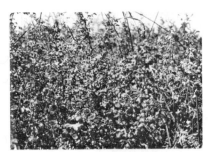

California rose. Photo courtesy East Bay Regional Park District Botanic Garden.

DOSAGE: For tea, use the standard dosage of one teaspoon of dried hips to one cup of hot water. When using fresh rose hips, put four in one cup of hot water: *We've got to cut down on some powerful herbs. Rose hips aren't going to hurt you.* For bites and stings, one application is enough.

Josephine uses the native species, not the domestic.

String beans are another one that can be used by diabetics. Eat string beans as a regular part of a meal.

When Josephine was growing up, there was no name for diabetes. Josephine thinks that what the locals called dropsy in the old days was actually diabetes.

Safflower

LATIN NAME: *Carthamus tinctorius*

NATIVE PLANT: No

PART USED: Top of plant, including the blossoms.

USE: Use as a moisturizer, and to treat cold sores, gout, and hypoglycemia. Contains a natural hydrochloric acid (utilizes sugar of fruits and oils). Neutralizes uric acid.

PREPARATION: Rub the oil on hands and skin as a moisturizer. When the oil is applied to cold sores, they dry in a few minutes. To treat gout, use as a soak. For preparation details, see the section on soaks in "Types of Medicinals."

For hypoglycemia, use the oil in general cooking: *I generally use safflower in the oil form in cooking, because I think you get all that out of the oil when you cook with it. They have safflower butter (oleo). You can get it out of that.*

DOSAGE: It seems to be safe no matter how much you take.

Josephine was unaware of safflower as a child. She believes she learned of its medicinal qualities from other Indian doctors. *I can never see where they can get safflower oil out of a safflower plant. They're always so dry-looking.*

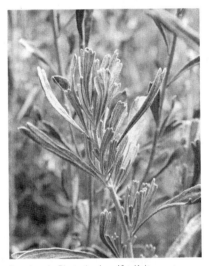

Sagebrush. Photo by Jennifer Kalt.

Sage

LATIN NAME: *Artemesia tridentata* (sagebrush)
Salvia apiana (obtained from "down south")
Salvia officinalis (commercial sage)

NATIVE PLANT: Yes, but not locally; also sold commercially.

PART USED: Leaves and stem

USE: Reduces fevers.

PREPARATION: Powder the leaves and steep as a tea, or purchase commercially. Alternatively, put the powder in ought capsules. To reduce fevers caused by measles in older children, put an even amount of sage and ginger (wild or commercial) in an ought capsule. This mixture can be useful in reducing other types of fevers in older children and adults as well. Never dispense to babies.

DOSAGE: Whenever you get a cold or fever, steep a quarter teaspoon in one cup of hot water for tea. Give only one capsule to older children. Adults may take one to three capsules at about two hour intervals until the fever breaks. Generally,

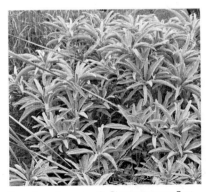

Sage from down south. Photo courtesy East Bay Regional Park District Botanic Garden.

only one or two capsules will be necessary: *When you take it, you watch the fever. If it's going down too slow, then you take another one. By the time they get two it'll be going down. Of course with the kids here, in a little while it'll go down.*

This tea is "*a hard one to take.*" Most people would rather have mountain balm. Sagebrush is a fine-leaved species that's mostly sticks: *We get them up towards Alturas. We don't have any sages growing around here... Different ones would bring it in, and we would always have it in seasoning... If we put it in stuffing, we ate it for two or three days* [laughs].

When Josephine and her siblings got fevers as children, they'd be given a tea of commercial sage and ginger. Sage of a different species is used inter-tribally for smudging: *They burn it in ceremonies to purify the house or run out the evil.* In northwest California Indian root is used for the same purpose.

Sagebrush, old (chaparral)

LATIN NAME: Unknown

NATIVE PLANT: Unknown

PART USED: Leaves and stem, without the flowers, because the flowers become "*soapy-like.*"

USE: Good for treating acne, boils, psoriasis and skin cancer.

PREPARATION: Use dry or fresh. To draw poisons out of the system, make a poultice by mashing up the leaves and mixing them with boiling water, enough to hold the leaves together. Apply a poultice or salve to acne, boils, psoriasis and skin cancer. For salve, use with wormwood leaves. For details on the preparation and use of poultices and salves, see the sections on poutices and salves in "Types of Medicinals."

DOSAGE: Apply as needed.

Chaparral has a "*funny, stink smell.*" *We call it old sagebrush.* It grows about two feet tall and has little leaves. Josephine believes she learned about it later in life from Ella Johnson, a respected basketry teacher, or someone else who lived in the area.

People used to put peroxide on their faces to treat acne. Witch hazel will do the same thing.

See also: wormwood.

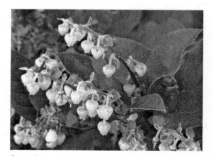

Salal. Photo by Jennifer Kalt.

Salal

KARUK NAME: purithkam'ippa(ha) ["huckleberry-side-bush"]

LATIN NAME: *Gaultheria shallon*

NATIVE PLANT: Yes

PART USED: Berries

USE: Food

PREPARATION: Eat berries raw or make into jelly.

DOSAGE: N/A

Josephine learned to eat salal berries from a member of the Hoopa Valley Tribe.

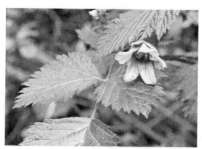

Salmonberry. Photo by Jennifer Kalt.

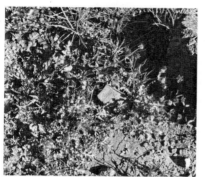

Purple sanicle. Photo courtesy East Bay Regional Park District Botanic Garden.

Salmonberry

LATIN NAME: *Rubus spectabilis*

NATIVE PLANT: Yes

PART USED: Berries

USE: Food

PREPARATION: Eat salmonberries raw. They will *"mush right up."*

DOSAGE: N/A

Sanicle, purple

KARUK NAME: ishmúchchah

LATIN NAME: *Sanicula bipinnatifida*

NATIVE PLANT: Yes

PART USED: Stem and leaves.

USE: Tumors (any kind of growth), ulcers, external wounds.

PREPARATION: For tumors and ulcers, steep one teaspoon to one cup of hot water. For poultice for external wounds, use fresh or dry. For preparation and use details, see the section on poultices in "Types of Medicinals."

DOSAGE: Drink the tea twice a day. For ulcers, drink the tea for three days, then stop for three days. Continue with this cycle for four to six weeks.

Purple sanicle has become rare in the local area, so Josephine doesn't use it much. She prefers blood root for tumors.

Sarsaparilla

LATIN NAME: *Smilax officinalis*

NATIVE PLANT: No

PART USED: Root

USE: Contains male hormone. Use as an antidote for mushroom or food poisoning. Good for rheumatism and gout. Also good for psoriasis.

PREPARATION: Dry and pulverize the root. Steep as a tea. For psoriasis, prepare as a salve. For preparation and use details, see the section on salves in "Types of Medicinals."

DOSAGE: Use one teaspoon to one cup of hot water. For a poison antidote, drink two to three cups at one sitting. For rheumatism and gout, take two times a day, and your aches and pains will be gone.

Josephine learned about sarsaparilla later in life. She has its brown root shipped in. Although others may use sarsaparilla for gout, Josephine uses the sap from wild grape for this purpose.

Sarsaparilla comes in from over around Mississippi and the lower states... I think it grows clear up through Georgia... We'd get it and have it at home. It'll be all rolled and dried... We used to just bite it off and chew it [laughs]. We just did it to be eating it. Of course, after I grew up and had the strokes, my uncle used to take me to Mount Shasta to the Chinese doctor, to Robert. That's when I'd get all that good stuff [laughs]. *He'd give me different things.*

See also: grape, wild.

Sassafras

LATIN NAME: *Sassifras albidum*

NATIVE PLANT: No

PART USED: Root

USE: Toothache and varicose ulcers (veins).

PREPARATION: For toothache, chew on a small piece to soften, then hold it where needed. Make a poultice for varicose ulcers (caused by the veins breaking and becoming sores). The root comes dried and rolled up. First, pound it, put boiling water on it to get it wet, then apply it with medical-supply tape so it'll stay. Leave it two or three days, if it will stay that long, then pull it off.

DOSAGE:Although this plant can be used for eyewashes and for congestion, it can be dangerous when made into a tea, so this isn't recommended.

Josephine acquired this plant by trading with other Indian doctors, including Ellis Lupe: *You've got to get this from back east... This comes from further up: Hampshire and Vermont and all of those states in there.* Sassafras will stain cloth orange.

Seaweed

LATIN NAME: Various

NATIVE PLANT: Yes, a different species for each use.

PART USED: Leaves

USE: These iodine-rich plants are good for goiters, thyroid, nails and hair loss: *It'll make them grow back good. You eat a lot of that, your hair will never turn gray. It stays black. And this is a new one they found—it cleanses radiation. If you have radiation treatments, it'll help build your body back up.*

For sore throats, gargle with the dark green species. For weight reduction, eat Irish moss, the white seaweed with purple edges that grows along the northerly coast of California. For food, harvest the species that grows on rocks two feet tall and a foot-and-a-half across.

PREPARATION: For goiter, thyroid, nails and hair loss eat raw seaweed daily, or dry it and eat it. Alternatively, fry it in bacon grease before eating (see below). For sore throat, make a gargle. For preparation details, see the section on gargles in "Types of Medicinals." For weight reduction, eat fresh or dried.

For food, gather the whole plant in May during low tides. For details about the gathering, drying, storing and cooking of seaweed, see the seaweed section in "Native Plant Foods."

DOSAGE: For goiter, thyroid, nails and hair loss eat quantities. For weight reduction eat the equivalent of 1-1/2 inches of dried seaweed twice a day. Take until you reach the desired weight.

Josephine learned about seaweed's use for weight reduction by trying it herself. She doesn't recall the source of her other medicinal knowledge about it: *We never had it inland. We used to get it on the coast when I lived there... When I went to Queto, Ecuador, I took a lot of it* [seaweed]. *Down there every little kid, and all the people, have these great big goiters. You see them walking around with big growths. I guess they had no salt. No iodine. They have to go clear back up to the Gulf of Mexico to get salt.*

Josephine was able to return a foster child with goiter to good health and color with seaweed. She fried and served it to the youngster for a year.

Josephine eats dried kelp. Kelp pills from Japan or China are now available for goiter.

Shepherd's purse (St. James weed)

KARUK NAME: chantinnihiich ["imitation-ticks"]

LATIN NAME: *Capsella bursa-pastoris*

NATIVE PLANT: No, but locally naturalized in yards.

PART USED: Top of the plant, including flowers when in bloom.

USE: Bleeding ulcers, hemorrhage after childbirth, and diarrhea.

PREPARATION: Gather by cutting off the top of the plant. Use fresh or dried. Pour boiling water over the plant tops. Steep one half hour, then strain. It will gel once the water becomes cold. *It's just like taking jello.* [...] *It turns to a white, thick slime after it's been put in hot water. Of course, that gel will seal wherever is bleeding.*

DOSAGE: It takes an indeterminate number of plants to create the gel, which appears to be located in the tiny, heart-shaped fruits (capsules). The casual observer can easily mistake these green-colored fruits for leaves.

For bleeding ulcers, make a quart, so the patient will keep drinking it. Stuff half a quart's worth of shepherd's purse tops into a quart-sized canning jar. Pour boiling water atop this, then follow the directions above to create the gel. Drink until the bleeding stops. For hemorrhage after childbirth, do the same.

The gel can be safely consumed in large quantities.

Josephine recalls an elder midwife using this plant: *A long time ago, we lost a lot of women in childbirth.*

Skullcap

LATIN NAME: Probably a *Penstemon*, based on a pressed plant specimen labeled by Josephine as skullcap

NATIVE PLANT: Yes, and other species also sold commercially.

PART USED: Leaves and stem.

USE: Neurotonic for epilepsy and fits.

PREPARATION: Mix with mistletoe and white lady slipper for epilepsy.

DOSAGE: Withheld due to danger of harm if plant isn't properly used.

Found in serpentine soil, where whole populations of this plant have been destroyed due to overharvesting by unethical gatherers.

Of the species of penstemon that grow in the Klamath Ranges Floristic Province *(P. anguineus, P. azureus, P. azureus var. azureus, P. davidsonii var. davidsonii, P. deustus, P. deustus var. suffrutescens, P. filiformis, P. heterodoxus, P. heterodoxus var. heterodoxus, P. heterophyllus, P. heterophyllus var. heterophyllus, P. laetus, P. laetus var. sagittatus, P. newberryi, P. newberryi var. berryi, P. parvulus, P. procerus, P. procerus var. brachyanthus, P. procerus var. formosus, P. purpusii, P. rattanii, P. rattanii var. rattanii, P. roezlii, P. rupicola, P. speciosus,* and *P. tracyi,* none are identified as growing on serpentine soils, while *Scutellaria antirrhinoides* (blue lobelia) is recognized as doing so.

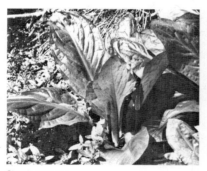

Skunk cabbage.
Photo by Deborah E. McConnell.

Skunk cabbage

LATIN NAME: *Lysichiton americanum*

NATIVE PLANT: Yes

PART USED: Leaves only.

USE: Treating tuberculosis. Relieving the pain of terminally ill patients, helping to ease them out emotionally.

PREPARATION: Steep as a tea.

DOSAGE: Use one teaspoon to one cup of hot water. For tuberculosis, drink one cup in the morning and one in the evening, or four half cups throughout the day. For pain, take as much as needed.

Skunk cabbage is a dangerous narcotic that should only be given when it's clear that a patient isn't going to make it.

Josephine learned about this plant from the old people: *In the early days there was a lot of TB in our area, and I saw them using it.*

Slippery elm

LATIN NAME: *Ulmus fulva*

NATIVE PLANT: No

PART USED: *There's a little button that comes out on the leaf. We use it just like we do the cottonwood shoots that come out in the spring.*

USE: Gargle with myrrh for bad breath, sore throat, and tonsillitis. When you feel a cold coming on, gargle with it to prevent sore throat.

PREPARATION: Boil water, then pour over the powdered form. For gargle, combine small amounts of slippery elm and myrrh. Alternatively, use these plants separately for sore throat and tonsillitis.

DOSAGE: Put about a quarter of a teaspoonful of powdered slippery elm and a "*pinch*" of myrrh in about a quarter of a cup of hot water. Make enough for two or three uses in a day. Note: It's possible to take too much myrrh, but myrrh is safe to use as a gargle with slippery elm. Do not swallow myrrh. For preparation and use details, see the section on gargles in "Types of Medicinals."

Josephine isn't sure when she first learned about slippery elm, but she thinks she learned about it at a doctor's gathering at Manitoba, Canada: *Of course, they've got it all over up in Canada. You can find it in the stores….My friend's up in there. He gets it. He comes down with all kinds of herbs* [laughs]. *He was coming down a couple times a year.*

See also: Myrrh and cottonwood.

Soapbrush (mountain laurel)

KARUK NAME: kithriip [-*ip*: "-bush"]

LATIN NAME: *Ceanothus integerrimus*

NATIVE PLANT: Yes

PART USED: Blossoms and shoots.

USE: Blossoms for soap. Pruned shoots for the warps in fine basketry.

PREPARATION: *We used to play with the blossoms when they were blooming to make soap out of it. We'd lather it up.* This is where Josephine's name for the plant comes from.

DOSAGE: N/A

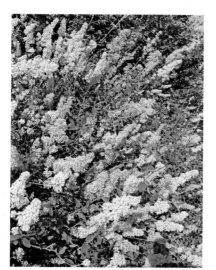

Soapbrush. Photo by Jennifer Kalt.

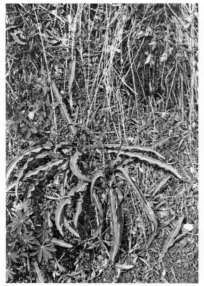

Soaproot. Photo by Deborah M. McConnell.

Soaproot

aka soap plant, a common name that Josephine does not use

KARUK NAME: imyúha ["layered-over"]

LATIN NAME: *Chlorogalum pomeridianum*

NATIVE PLANT: Yes

PART USED: Bulb

USE: Relieves itch caused by poison oak.

PREPARATION: Use the fresh bulbs. After digging them, wash off any dirt. Cut the bulbs in half and rub the flat (inside) portion up and down on the affected areas. If you run out of juice, quarter the bulb.

DOSAGE: Apply whenever the rash itches. Usually, one bulb will be sufficient to relieve the rash. In the wintertime, when the bulbs contain less juice, more will be needed.

The juice of the bulb has healing qualities. When firefighters or others come to Josephine with poison oak rash, she advises them not to scratch it, lest it spread, and provides them with, or tells them about, soaproot, or other of her poison oak remedies.

For more about poison oak remedies, *see also*: dandelion, manzanita, mullein, plantain, ribbed and wide-leaf, Solomon seal, walnut, black, wormwood (mugwort), and oatmeal and ocean water in the non-herbal cures section.

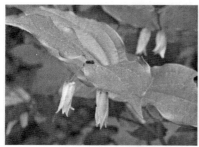

Starry Solomon's seal (*Smilacina stellata*). Photo by Sydney Carothers.

Smith's fairy bells (*Disporum smithii*). Photo by Jennifer Kalt.

Solomon seal

aka starry Solomon's seal, a common name that Josephine does not use

KARUK NAME: pikvassáhiich (fat Solomon's seal, *S. racemosa* var. *amplexicaulis*) ["imitation-plume"]

LATIN NAME: *Smilacina stellata*. Josephine uses false Solomon's seal (fat Solomon's seal) (*S. racemosa*) more rarely. Two pressed plant specimens labeled by Josephine as Solomon's seal are from the genus *Disporum*, probably *D. smithii* in one instance.

NATIVE PLANT: Yes

PART USED: Peanut-like "*bulbs*" on the root, red berries in the fall, or juice from the top of the plant, depending on the use.

USE: Bulbs and berries are given to women in labor. Its sedative qualities lessen pain during labor. It also coagulates the blood, stopping hemorrhaging after giving birth. The juice is used to prevent poison oak rash, heal bruised or broken bones, and draw out black and blue marks caused by blood beneath the skin, as with spikenard.

PREPARATION: Each plant has one (more rarely, two) small, peanut-sized bulbs. In the spring the bulb is small; as the plant gets older, the bulb gets bigger. Josephine usually uses the bulb fresh, although it can be dried. Soak dried bulbs in water prior to use.

Women in labor should hold a single bulb between their gums and teeth, and suck on it. In the fall use three to four berries in the same manner as a single bulb.

When the men who work in the woods get cut and bleed a lot, they break the whole stem off, and the juice will drain out. It's a slimy stuff that comes right out. It'll gel and stop the bleeding. While it's better to use the gel fresh for this purpose, you can also pound (powder) the dry stems and put the powder in an open wound to stop the bleeding. It works by coagulating the blood.

If you're out in the woods and you get poison oak on you, and you know where it hit you, then you go get that stuff [juice] *and put it on.*

Apply the juice to broken bones: *Sometimes your bone will break through the skin. That's when you use it… You cut this thing and get the juice out of it. It'll bleed in under the skin, and you've got to put it on there… Different ones here put that juice on it.*

The bulbs were used by the midwives of old. Because she's always been immune to poison oak, Josephine doesn't remember how she learned about this plant's qualities as a rash preventative.

For more about poison oak remedies, *see also:* dandelion, manzanita, mullein, plantain, ribbed and wide-leaf, soaproot, walnut, black, wormwood (mugwort), and oatmeal and ocean water in the non-herbal cures section.

Redwood sorrel. Photo by Jennifer Kalt.

Sorrel, redwood

KARUK NAME: takkánnaafich

LATIN NAME: *Oxalis oregana*

NATIVE PLANT: Yes

PART USED: Whole plant (roots, stems, and pink flowers).

USE: Makes penicillin for use on sprains, sore joints, sore muscles, arthritis, cuts, sores, and infected wounds.

PREPARATION: After gathering the plant, roots and all, rinse it clean. Stuff a gallon-sized crock with redwood sorrel. Bury the jar in a damp cool place in the ground, covering it with about a foot of soil. Leave it there for two or three months. When you remove the jar, it will be full of penicillin in the form of a fibrous material (gray mold). The plant itself turns black when it rots down. Take a clean stick and move it around in the crock to collect the fibers, and transfer these into another jar. Put alcohol purchased in a pharmacy, not rubbing alcohol, in with the black remainder.

DOSAGE: Use two tablespoons of alcohol per pint of rotted redwood sorrel. Rub this mixture two times a day on sprains, sore joints, pulled muscles and arthritis. If still hurting the next day, reapply. Lay the mold (penicillin) inside cuts and wounds and leave it in there. The mold will also stop the bleeding.

Redwood sorrel grows all over near the creeks. It grows all over your backyard. You've got all kind of medicines close by.

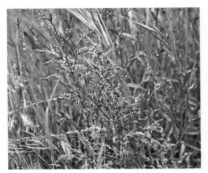

Sourgrass. Photo by Beverly Ortiz.

Sourgrass (sheep sorrel)

aka sheep's sorrel

LATIN NAME: *Rumex acetosella*

NATIVE PLANT: No, but locally naturalized.

PART USED: Top of plant.

USE: Jaundice, stomach ulcers (hemorrhage), excessive urination (diuretic), mouth cancer, skin tumors (dark moles on the skin and little lumps under the skin), boils.

PREPARATION: Steep "*a lot*" of sourgrass tops (stem, leaves, and reddish flower clusters) in hot water to make a tea for treating jaundice, stomach ulcers, hemorrhage. Can cause excessive urination. Use fresh or dried for tea. Chew fresh sourgrass to treat mouth cancers. Make a poultice of sourgrass tops dipped in hot water to treat skin tumors and boils: *You've got to dip it in hot water to get the stuff* [medicine] *to come out of it.*

DOSAGE: For the tea, use the standard teaspoon to one cup. Drink half a cup four times per day. Take for one week, stop for a week, then continue. For jaundice and stomach ulcers, take for three or four weeks. As a diuretic, take once.

Sorrel grows all over the valley and sides of the roads... We'd chew it up, eat it in the springtime... The leaves that come out of the ground are good to eat. You pick them before they start getting tough. They're shaped like little arrows, and that's what you put in your salads.

As with purslane, Josephine tried using sourgrass to loose weight, due to its diuretic properties: *When we wanted to lose a few pounds, we'd run out and get some and eat it, or cook it up and eat it* [laughs]. The reason: *Because you do nothing but urinate for about 24 hours* [laughs]... *Me and my girlfriends must have been crazy* [laughs]. *We'd do anything* [to loose weight].

When Josephine was young, a tea from the flowering tops of sourgrass was used for jaundice and stomach ulcers: *Jaundice is a disease of the liver. It's probably from eating stuff that wasn't cooked right, or was old, or something. It affected your liver... I think it was that sourness in the leaves that helped jaundice. You know if you put the sorrel tea in your mouth, it's going to pucker up inside your mouth. You can just feel it puckering. And I think that's what stops the hemorrhaging. You just drink it. It's gets in your stomach and puckers it up.*

Sheep sorrel poultices were commonly applied to skin and canker sores, the latter occurring because the old people constantly smoked pipes. In the latter situation, the leaves could be mashed, then applied.

Spearmint

LATIN NAME: *Mentha spicata* var. *spicata*

NATIVE PLANT: No

PART USED: The upper part of the plant, including the flowers when in bloom.

USE: For sour stomach (gas pain) and baby colic. Add for taste to liquid goldenseal and blood root teas.

PREPARATION: Use fresh or dried. Steep as a tea for stomach trouble.

The decision to add spearmint for taste to liquid medicinals, and how much to add, depends on the individual. When using capsules, it's unnecessary to add any mint.

DOSAGE: Steep one teaspoon in one cup of hot water. You can drink spearmint tea everyday with no ill effect.

For sour stomach, take once a day. For baby colic dispense seven to ten drops from a baby dropper, depending on the size drops. One dose should be enough: *If you get gas in your stomach, like babies get colic, just put a few drops in their water and let them suck on it, or just spoon it to them... Elder people who have gas and sour stomachs can drink half a cup.*

See also: ginger, goldenseal, and blood root.

Spikenard

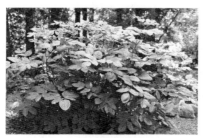

Spikenard. Photo courtesy East Bay Regional Park District Botanic Garden.

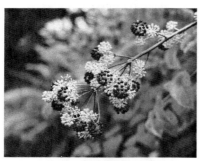

Spikenard, detail. Photo courtesy East Bay Regional Park District Botanic Garden.

Recalls Josephine: *We used to call it bear berry.*

LATIN NAME: *Aralia californica*

NATIVE PLANT: Yes

PART USED: Root

USE: Drains the sinuses. Good for sore throat and canker sores. Good for stroke symptoms, draws blood from bruises and black eyes, and relives swelling from sore joints (including the shoulder), and arthritis. Also good for "female problems" (excessive menstruation and menstrual pain).

PREPARATION: To dry, split the root and lay it with the centers facing up. For sinuses, put tea up nose, like salt water. For sore throat, gargle with a strong tea. For preparation details, see the section on gargles in "Types of Medicinals." For canker sores, hold it in your mouth and rinse as you would with any antiseptic. For stroke victims, apply poultice to the back of the head and neck, clear down to the tail bone, and let the patient lie in it. For bruises, black eyes, sore joints, and arthritis make poultice, which draws out blood from beneath the skin (blood clots). For female problems, make into a douche.

DOSAGE: For nose drops, use the standard teaspoon to one cup of water. Put drops in nose twice a day. Gargle two or three times a day to treat sore throat.

Hold spikenard against canker sores for two minutes before rinsing, three or four times a day.

For a douche, steep about half a cup of the root in a half-gallon of hot water. Douche once a day.

This plant, which is in the ginseng family, has a distinctive smell: *You can smell it all over when you pick that stuff... The old midwives used it all the time... I had a stroke when I was rather young, in my thirties. I was in a coma. This old lady sent my neighbor out to get some. [She] told them to mash it up. She came in, and she poulticed it down the back of my head clear down my spine. I laid in it all night. The next afternoon I came out of it. My mind was pretty clear. I was mad at the doctor. I said, "Why didn't you let me go?" [laughs]. I didn't want to drag around. I had one before, and it took me so long to get over it.*

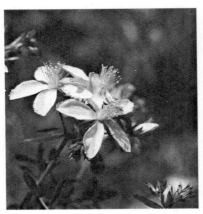

St. John's wort. Photo by Beverly Ortiz.

St. John's wort (Klamath weed)

KARUK NAME: (i)thivthaneentáayvar pinishxanahyâachas ["earth-spoiler" "quite-long-plants"]

LATIN NAME: *Hypericum perforatum*

NATIVE PLANT: No, but locally naturalized.

PART USED: Black glands on edges of petals, with petals included.

USE: Settling the stomach during such illnesses as stomach flu and HIV/AIDS: *That way they can hold the food down.* [. . . .] *I give that to my patients when they get really sick, like my cancer patients…* Also a relaxant, used to treat nervousness related to Parkinson's Disease.

PREPARATION: *I wait until the petals start to dry down, and then pick the heads of the flowers off.* Depending on the weather, the petals dry down as early as June. In the mountains this occurs as late as August. Josephine snips the flower heads into a paper bag. She lays them out to dry at home. *The flower has tiny stems that come up, and it's got little black things on top. I've got to pick the whole flower, but I wait until the petal part dies down, and keep that little inside part. I use the petal, too, because it isn't going to do any harm.*

DOSAGE: Use the standard ratio of one teaspoonful to one cup of hot water. Start with just half a cup to see how your system will react. *If* [a patient's body] *rejects it, then you give them something else. A lot of people can't take the same herb.*

For settling the stomach: *I make a tea and have them drink it half an hour before they eat anything.* For Parkinson's Disease, take two cups per day. It's okay to take daily.

A long time ago they'd give [St. John's wort] *to people with cancer, and it would settle their stomach, just like the peach leaves.* Locals gathered it by the paper bagfuls and stored it. *We had a lot of it in the area. It used to just take over the hay fields and everything… They brought in some kind of a Japanese beetle one time to try to kill it all… They cleaned it out, but it's coming back.*

See also: peach, domestic.

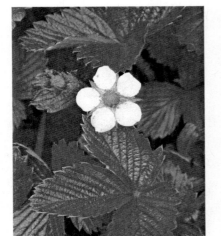

Wild strawberry. Photo by Jennifer Kalt.

Strawberry, wild

LATIN NAME: *Fragaria vesca*

NATIVE PLANT: Yes

PART USED: Medicinals: Fresh leaves. Food: Fruit.

USE: Any type of mouth sore, including canker sores and gum boils, and sore throat. Also food.

PREPARATION: Always use the leaves fresh. These are particularly good for canker sores. For sore throat, use fresh leaves to make a gargle. For preparation details, see the section on gargles in "Types of Medicinals." Gather and eat wild strawberries onsite, when fresh.

DOSAGE: For sores and boils, chew on the fresh leaves as often as needed. Steep a teaspoon in half a cup of water. For sore throat, gargle two to three times a day. Repeat the next day if sore throat persists.

Josephine has always known about strawberry leaves.

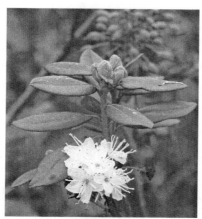

Swamp tea. Photo by Jennifer Kalt.

Swamp tea (Labrador tea)

Some locals use the name "coast tea."

LATIN NAME: *Ledum glandulosum*

NATIVE PLANT: Yes

PART USED: Leaves with some stems.

USE: High blood pressure.

PREPARATION: Drink as a tea, but make it fresh each time: *It's like the peach leaves, it builds up a toxic poison if you leave it sit.*

DOSAGE: Make in the standard dosage of one teaspoon to one cup of hot water, but only drink half a cup, once in the morning and once in the evening. Drink for no more than three days. Since care must be taken not to drink too much over a long period of time, Josephine recommends against drinking this tea recreationally.

Tanoak

KARUK NAME: xunyêep ["acorn-soup-good-tree"]

LATIN NAME: *Lithocarpus densiflorus*

NATIVE PLANT: Yes

PART USED: Acorns and bark.

USE: Poultice for burns. Eyewash for eye infections and cataracts. Food.

PREPARATION: For treating burns, use unleached flour or burn pieces of oak in the heater stove and save the ashes. For treating eye infections and cataracts, retain the first batch of acorn-leaching water. For preparation details, see "Oak." For details on the gathering and preparation of acorns for flour and food, see the acorn subsection in the nuts section of "Native Plant Foods."

DOSAGE: For dosage details, *see also* Oak.

Tanoak. Photo by Jennifer Kalt

The tannin in tanoaks is useful for treating severe burns. Tanoak acorn soup can strengthen a person: *When people are sick, acorn builds their strength. I make a lot of acorn for people that are ailing. They can hold it down, whereas they can't hold other food down... With boys that are wrassling and running, you give them acorns to build up their strength. We use the alder bark to make a tea that strengthens their lungs... I took it for a while because my lungs were bad...a couple of years ago* [ca. 1999]... *A long time ago, they used to have marathons. They ran for miles, and they always took that. They'd give them acorns, and then alder bark tea.* Although the long-distance running and marathons of old no longer occur, and the use of alder bark tea has been largely discontinued, wrestling still occurs, and acorn soup is still used to build the strength of the participants, including some of Josephine's nephews.

See also: alder, white. For an alternative burn remedy, *see also*: manzanita.

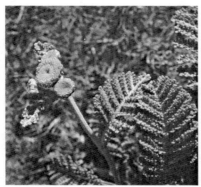

Tansy. Photo by Beverly Ortiz.

Tansy

LATIN NAME: Probably *Tanacetum camphoratum*

NATIVE PLANT: Yes

PART USED: Flower

USE: Reduces fevers.

PREPARATION: Steep as a tea.

DOSAGE: Watch dosage carefully. Use in small quantities, about a shot glassful.

The old people preferred yarrow for reducing fevers, but used tansy if yarrow was unavailable. Josephine doesn't use tansy; she prefers other fever remedies.

See also: yarrow.

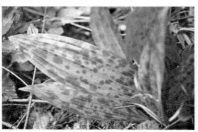

TB flower. Photo courtesy East Bay Regional Park District Botanic Garden.

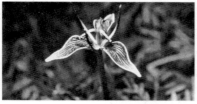

TB flower, detail. Photo courtesy East Bay Regional Park District Botanic Garden.

TB flower (skunk lily)

LATIN NAME: *Scoliopus bigelovii*

NATIVE PLANT: Yes

PART USED: Leaves

USE: Good for tuberculosis and lung ailments.

PREPARATION: Use leaves fresh or dried. Dry upside down, crush leaves, and store in a gallon jar. Steep as a tea.

DOSAGE: Put two heaping tablespoons of crushed skunk lily leaves in a pot. Pour hot water onto the leaves, filling the pot. Cover and steep for twenty minutes. Drink one cup in the morning and evening, or four half cups throughout the day.

Skunk lily has yellow flowers.

Josephine learned about this plant from the old people: *In the early days there was a lot of TB in our area, and I saw them using it.*

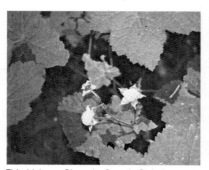

Thimbleberry. Photo by Beverly Ortiz.

Thimbleberry

LATIN NAME: *Rubus parviflorus*

NATIVE PLANT: Yes

PART USED: Berries

USE: Food

PREPARATION: Since the berries are mushy, eat them raw, as soon as they're gathered.

DOSAGE: N/A

Thistle, milk

LATIN NAME: *Silybum marianum*

NATIVE PLANT: No, but locally naturalized.

PART USED: Sap

USE: Used for warts, like castor oil.

PREPARATION: Cut stem and collect the milky sap.

DOSAGE: Apply two times a day.

Josephine remembers milk thistle's use for warts during her childhood.

Milk thistle didn't exist in the Hoopa area until the 1940s, when hay was imported for animal feed. Star thistle was imported the same way.

A field where milk thistle once grew was paved over. It also used to grow on a nearby creek bar. Today Josephine obtains hers in a health food store.

Tobacco, Eastern

LATIN NAME: *Nicotiana* sp. *Nicotiniana tabacum* is the cultivated species.

NATIVE PLANT: No

PART USED: Leaf

USE: Toothache. (Indian tobacco is too powerful to be used for this purpose.)

PREPARATION: Use fresh or dried. Put a "*wad*" of eastern tobacco around your tooth, and hold it there to deaden the pain.

DOSAGE: Use a small amount. As Josephine puts it: *Wad up a little piece.*

Eastern tobacco grew in the local area prior to the building of roads for automobiles.

Josephine's father grew eastern tobacco and chewed it all his life. Although his teeth were worn, he never had a toothache. The seeds of the eastern tobacco may have been brought to the local area by Josephine's paternal grandfather, who came from the east, or by her Abenaki great-great-grandfather.

Josephine used to grow eastern tobacco in the 1960s. She also obtained eastern tobacco from fields and drying sheds located near West Point.

Tobacco, Indian

KARUK NAME: ihêeraha ["being smoked"]

LATIN NAME: *Nicotiana quadrivalvis* (synonym *N. bigelovii*)

NATIVE PLANT: Yes

PART USED: Leaves

USE: Relaxant.

PREPARATION: *We just pull the bottom leaves off and save the rest to go to seed. It won't come up if you spread the seeds.* Dry the leaves.

DOSAGE: Dosage withheld due to concern about overuse.

The species of Indian tobacco used for this purpose has small, cream-colored, trumpet-shaped flowers. It grows in the mountains and was used in a variety of "*old medicine.*" Josephine's grandmother smoked Indian tobacco before she went to bed to relax, as did the men who worked for the family putting in the hay crop and cutting the winter wood supply. The workers smoked it when they went to bed. One Indian tobacco locale was destroyed when non-Indians pulled the plants up by the roots.

Toyon (holly berry, Christmas berry)

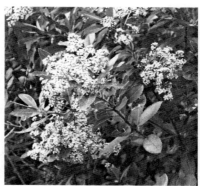
Toyon. Photo by Jennifer Kalt.

KARUK NAME: pasyîip

LATIN NAME: *Heteromeles arbutifolia*

NATIVE PLANT: Yes

PART USED: Berries

USE: Childhood entertainment.

PREPARATION: Children used to roast the berries in the fall for a treat. They held a branch with berries over the fire, "*twisting it around*" to ensure even roasting.

DOSAGE: N/A

Josephine once tried roasted holly berries, but did not like them.

Valerian

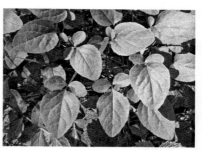
Valerian (*Valerian* sp.). Photo by Jennifer Kalt.

LATIN NAME: *Valeriana sitchensis*

NATIVE PLANT: Yes

PART USED: Stem and leaves.

USE: Promotes sleep. Used for symptoms of restlessness (headache, muscle twitching, and spasms): *You take it when you feel different things, a lot of times at night. When you overdo and get cramps in your legs and feet, you take it. It's a relaxer...*

PREPARATION: Use fresh or dried. Steep as a tea.

DOSAGE: Valerian has narcotic qualities, and you can get addicted to it, so use it sparingly. Use the standard teaspoon to one cup of hot water. Take half a cup three times per day.

Josephine learned about valerian from the old people: *We've always had it grow-ing all around up at Somes Bar... I don't know about the ones that they use in Hoopa, but we always had plenty of it. It grows where the banks are damp. Where there's a lot of moisture.* In 2004 Josephine discovered that a whole hillside of valerian had been cleaned out by some unknown, unprincipled gatherer.

See also: vervain.

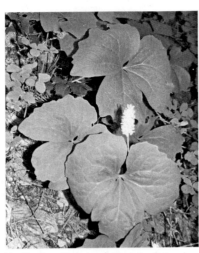

Vanilla plant (*Achyls* sp.). Photo by Deborah E. McConnell.

Vanilla plant

LATIN NAME: *Achlys californica*

NATIVE PLANT: Yes

PART USED: Stems and leaves.

USE: Insect repellent.

PREPARATION: Hang vanilla plants in closet or put into drawers to repel insects. You can also make a candle for the same purpose. For instructions on making the candle, *see:* lemon mint.

DOSAGE: N/A

Achlys californica is one of two species of vanilla plant used by Josephine. It is unknown whether the second species of *Achlys* that grows in California, *A. triphylla* var. *triphylla*, is Josephine's second vanilla plant.

See also: lemon mint.

Vervain

LATIN NAME: Unknown. Possibly *Verbena lasiostachys*, which grows in the Klamath Ranges (*The Jepson Manual* on-line).

NATIVE PLANT: Unknown

PART USED: Stem and leaves.

USE: Pain killer, irrespective of species.

PREPARATION: Use fresh or dried. Steep as a tea.

DOSAGE: Vervain has narcotic qualities, and you can get addicted to it, so use it sparingly. As with other herbal medicines, Josephine recommends that, at first, an adult take only about a quarter cup of vervain to find out whether or not they're allergic to it: *Just take a little, and see what it's going to do to you.*

Since vervain is stronger than valerian, it should be taken in smaller dosages. Prepare the tea using the standard ratio of a teaspoon of herb to one cup of hot water, but only drink about a quarter of a cup two times per day, and, at most, three-quarters of a cup.

See also: valerian.

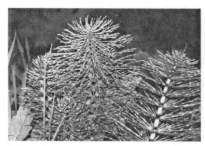

Wahoo. Photo by Beverly Ortiz.

Wahoo (horsetail)

LATIN NAME: *Equisetum telmateia* ssp. *braunii*

NATIVE PLANT: Yes

PART USED: Young shoots.

USE: Primarily used as a diuretic. Good for strengthening hair and toughening nails. Dissolves kidney stones. Used to remove phlegm from an infant's throat. High in silica.

PREPARATION: For a diuretic effect, eat the "*really, really tender shoots*" fresh as the plant comes out of the ground. Cook them like asparagus: *When it first comes up it's tender, and you cook it. If it gets too big, it's tough. You can't eat it. It's like eating kelp. Kelp helps your hair.*

Horsetail is steeped as a tea to promote hair growth and stout nails, as well as dissolve kidney stones. When horsetail has grown about seven or eight inches tall in the spring, before it forms side-branches, Josephine cuts off four of the stalks and dries them for later use.

When babies with whooping cough and colds can't cough up the phlegm, rinse the stem with water and put its growing tip down into the baby's throat. Gently twirl it around in the infant's throat to catch the phlegm, then draw out the stalk and phlegm.

DOSAGE: For a diuretic, eat twice a day.

For tea, steep the standard teaspoon to one cup of hot water. For promoting hair growth and strong nails, drink the tea two times a day for a week.

For dissolving kidney stones, drink the tea three times a day. You've got to make it stronger than the gooseberry, and it takes a little longer, because the gooseberry has that acid in it that'll eat the stone up. You've probably got to take the horsetail about four or five weeks, but the gooseberry will dissolve it in two days.

Horsetail looks "*like asparagus*": *It comes up where it's wet. It's a little spike thing.* Josephine began to eat it, under the instruction of a Yurok elder, after moving to the Hoopa Valley. *Grandma was Down River. Yurok.*

The silica-rich stems of horsetail were used as a type of sandpaper "*a long time ago*": *The old people talked about it. I never did try it.* In the past, Josephine also saw older people use horsetail as a tea for whooping cough and colds.

See also: gooseberry and kelp.

Wallflower

LATIN NAME: *Erysimum capitatum* var. *capitatum*

NATIVE PLANT: Yes

PART USED: Whole upper part of the plant, including the flowers, but never the root.

USE: Abortifacient

PREPARATION: Withheld

DOSAGE: Withheld

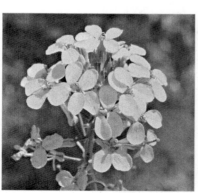

Wallflower. Photo by Jennifer Kalt.

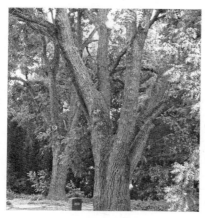

Black walnut. Photo courtesy East Bay Regional Park District Botanic Garden.

Walnut, black

KARUK NAME: apxantich'athithxuntapan'íppa(ha) (*walnut, J.* sp.) ["whiteman-hazel-tree"]

LATIN NAME: Probably *Juglans californica* var. *hindsii*

NATIVE PLANT: Yes, but not locally.

PART USED: Hull

USE: Kills parasites and worms. Used for poison oak and other rashes.

PREPARATION: For parasites and worms, steep as a tea. For poison oak and other rashes, make a wash; it will stain your skin.

DOSAGE: For parasites and worms, drink a quarter of a cup once a day for two days at most. *Now we use goldenseal for parasites and worms. Even the dog. Take a big* [double ought] *capsule full.*

For rashes, wash periodically with a strong, warm tea. For preparation details, see the section on washes in "Types of Medicinals."

Josephine recalls that the walnuts at the Old Home Place, which grew along the sled road, were thick shelled. She speculates that her "*old grandpa*" probably planted them when he came.

Avoid eating walnuts before they've dried, lest you develop diarrhea and mouth sores: *Then we'd go get the raspberry leaves, and pick and eat them.* Josephine notes that some people use walnut for dying gray willow sticks and, for decoration, the hazel around the top of hazel-handle and clothing baskets. She has used it herself to dye gray willow sticks, but uses commercial dye for her handle baskets. For dye, soak basketry material in cold water for several days in a hull dye bath in a long tub. Although the older generation sometimes dyed their hair with walnut to eliminate the gray, Josephine does not recommend this, as the hair will turn green.

See also: goldenseal and raspberry. For more about poison oak remedies, see also: dandelion, manzanita, mullein, plantain, ribbed and wide-leaf, soaproot, Solomon seal, wormwood (mugwort), and oatmeal and ocean water in the non-herbal cures section.

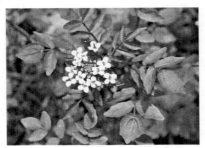

Watercress. Photo by Jennifer Kalt.

Watercress

LATIN NAME: *Rorippa nasturtium-aquaticum*

NATIVE PLANT: No, but locally naturalized.

PART USED: Top of the plants before they flower.

USE: Mostly used for food. A long time ago, watercress was taken for scurvy.

PREPARATION: Clip (prune) watercress before it blooms, after which it gets woody. Watercress will regrow when clipped. Use fresh in salads or boil like spinach: *We used to put vinegar on it* [when cooked]. [….] *Whatever kind we had.*

DOSAGE: For scurvy, eat as much of the fresh plant as you can until you are cured.

Watercress has a hot, peppery flavor. At the Old Home Place where Josephine grew up, watercress was plentiful in a pond created by nearby hydraulic mining operations. It also grew in the ditch the family used to irrigate their garden: *We'd go down and pick it, and mother would cook it. We'd put it in salads… Down in the ponds our old cows used to get in…and tramp it all down, because they ate it too… We tried to fence them out.* The fence consisted of wooden poles, but the cows managed to get access to the pond from another nearby field. They'd wade into the pond to eat it.

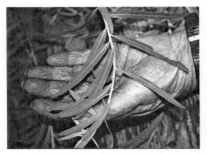

Gray willow. Photo by Beverly Ortiz.

Willow, gray

KARUK NAME: pâarak

LATIN NAME: *Salix exigua* (synonym *S. hindsiana*)

NATIVE PLANT: Yes

PART USED: Leaves

USE: Treating moles that can become cancerous, canker sores, and blood poison. Also for treating rheumatism.

PREPARATION: Peel off the leaves by running your hand along the shoots, starting at the tip. Use the leaves fresh or dried. Mash fresh leaves until they become paste-like. Crumble dried leaves and add just enough boiling water to cover them. Apply the paste, then wrap to make a poultice. Alternatively, for moles and canker sores, apply with a commercial bandage. Reapply daily. For preparation details, see the section on poultices in "Types of Medicinals."

DOSAGE: Reapply daily until healed. About one particular case of rheumatism in the knee of "one old fellow," Josephine recalls: [W]e *just put the whole plant, leaves and stems, and everything on his knee. At nighttime, we put it* [the poultice] *on and kept it damp. Put a hot water bottle on it, and it will stay moist and warm. Use it about three days and make a new one.* In this case, the knee was poulticed for about a week.

Local weavers use peeled gray willow shoots for basketry warp. While Josephine always knew about gray willow poultices, she used peppernut instead: *If you're in an area where there's no peppernuts, then you can use this one. But when we have peppernuts, we use them… Peppernuts are a lot stronger. They'll draw faster.*

See also: peppernuts.

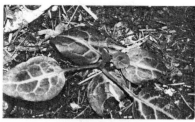

Wintermint. Photo by Deborah E. McConnell.

Wintermint

aka wintergreen, a common name that Josephine does not use

KARUK NAME: yumaaréempeeshara ["dead-person's-best-trail"]

LATIN NAME: *Pyrola picta*

NATIVE PLANT: Yes

PART USED: Leaves, stem, and flowers.

USE: Bladder problems that result from bad kidneys.

PREPARATION: Steep as a tea.

DOSAGE: Use the standard teaspoon to one cup of hot water, or, if you wish, make the tea a little stronger. Take half a cup four times daily until bladder problems gone.

This plant looks like pipsissewa and is used for the same purposes. Josephine has always known about it. The Karuk name derives from the use of this plant as a "medicine for a child who is sick, 'looking like a dead person'" (Schenck and Gifford 1952:387).

See also: pipsissewa.

Witch grass

LATIN NAME: Unknown

NATIVE PLANT: No

PART USED: Blades

USE: Expels worms in dogs.

PREPARATION: N/A

DOSAGE: N/A

Dogs eat the young blades of witch grass, an annual, to expel worms. It grows by Josephine's chicken house.

Wood betony

LATIN NAME: Unknown

NATIVE PLANT: Unknown

PART USED: Root

USE: Indigestion, stomach cramps, worms, Parkinson's disease, and jaundice from taking drugs

PREPARATION: Use fresh or dried. Use the standard teaspoon to one cup of hot water.

DOSAGE: This plant has no inherent danger associated with its use. For indigestion caused by bloating from eating too much, take one cupful with a little peppermint added. For stomach cramps, also take one cupful.

For worms take one cupful, then wait three to four days and take another cupful. *The eggs won't wash out until four days later. You've got to take it again to get rid of that...*

If you've got Parkinson's Disease, you've got to take it pretty much every day...
You've got to take it for jaundice a good five or six weeks...

Josephine obtains wood betony from an Indian doctor in Kansas. The plant, which grows on river bars and has a yellow stalk, looks similar to turkey mullein, but doesn't grow as tall. It has a spongy, white root. Josephine has been aware of its healing properties all of her life. For indigestion Josephine prefers to use mint teas, which are more readily available.

See also: catnip, peppermint, and spearmint.

Wormwood (mugwort)

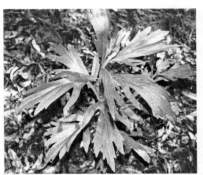

Wormwood. *A. douglasiana.*
Photo by Deborah E. McConnell.

KARUK NAME: káat (*A. douglasiana*)

LATIN NAME: *Artemesia douglasiana* (mugwort)
Artemisia ludoviciana subsp. *ludoviciana* (wormwood)

NATIVE PLANT: Yes. Use both species interchangeably.

PART USED: Leaves and their stems. Dried flowers for salves.

USE: Tick repellent and lice treatment. Used to treat liver trouble (swollen liver, as with jaundice); clean drugs and alcohol out of the system; treat sore throats and tonsillitis; and prevent and treat colds. Used, as well, to treat bruised and swollen limbs (sprains, arthritis, sore knees). In fact, Josephine considers wormwood to be the best herbal medicine for sprains. Also used to treat skin cancer, yeast infections, poison oak rash, and diabetics whose feet turn color. Used to treat sores that don't heal (skin sores, cancerous, bedsores), and ulcerated sores and skin diseases, such as psoriasis, scabies, mange, ringworm, acne and boils.

PREPARATION: To repel ticks, rub the fresh leaves on your clothes, near the ankles, along the waistline, on your sleeves, and at the back of the neck. You can also rub it directly on your skin. *When we go out and pick sticks, like hazel sticks, or pick up acorns, we just rub it on our arms and legs, and it keeps the ticks off.* For lice, prepare as a rinse. For preparation details, see the section on rinses for hair in "Types of Medicinals."

For liver trouble, steep as a tea to drink. To clean drugs and alcohol out of the system, also steep as a tea.

For sore throats and tonsillitis, or if you feel a cold coming on, steep as a tea to gargle. For more details, see the section on gargles in "Types of Medicinals."

For chest colds, make a poultice with wormwood: *When you get chest colds, you dip it in hot water, put it on, and wrap it.*

For bruises and swelling (sprains and arthritis), poultice wormwood or soak in it. For knee problems, wrap a poultice of the leaves around the affected area. Keep heat on it mostly at night using a hot water bottle or heating pad.

For skin cancer, apply a poultice of the leaves: *At nighttime, it's best to make a bed of the leaves, put it between a piece of cloth, and wrap it with plastic to keep it damp.*

For details on the preparation and use of poultices, see the section on poultices in "Types of Medicinals."

For yeast infections, make a soak or wash, depending on the affected area. For yeast infections under the breast and poison oak rash make a wash.

When poison oak rash is severe, pour wormwood solution, while the water is warm, over the entire body while standing in a bathtub. For posterior yeast infections and arthritis make a soak. Josephine considers wormwood to be the best treatment for yeast infections: *You can get wormwood and make a strong tea and it will last a week. Just keep warming it up, and put your hands in it.*

For ones that have diabetes really bad, where the feet turn color, we use wormwood and Jimson weed for soaking. We use the Jimson weed with the purple stem... The ones with the purple stem are kind of bushy and stay close to the ground... I think it kills the pain in your feet. For details on the preparation and use of soaks and rinses, see the sections on soaks and rinses in "Types of Medicinals."

Make a salve with coltsfoot, Johnny-jump-up (violet), and heal-all for sores that don't heal (skin sores, cancerous sores, bedsores). Make a salve with colts-foot, plantain, and garden violet (if pain) for boils, ulcerated sores, and skin diseases, like psoriasis, scabies, mange, and ringworm. Make a salve with old sagebrush for acne, boils, psoriasis and skin cancer.

Josephine used *A. leudoviciana* subsp. *leudoviciana* the day she made salves with project contributors. She also sends people to the coast to obtain *A. doug-lasiana* for medicinal purposes. For details on the preparation and use of salves, see the section on salves in "Types of Medicinals."

DOSAGE: For lice, make a fresh gallon of the rinse each time, using half as much leaves as water.

Wormwood isn't harmful when used externally, but can be if taken internally: *A lot of the old Indians I remember used to take it internally, but it's not good to do that. It burns your kidneys out* [if you overdo it]. *It's got a lot of camphor in it...*

Make wormwood tea in the standard dosage of a teaspoon to one cup of hot water. For liver trouble, take about half a cup twice a day for two days, then quit and don't take it again. *You can take it maybe a day or two for jaundice...*

To clean drugs and alcohol out of the system, also take half a cup. Don't take internally for more than three days, due to potential harm to the kidneys.

For sore throat, tonsillitis, or if you feel a cold coming on, gargle three times a day with as strong and hot a tea as you can tolerate. When poulticing chest colds, keep poultice on overnight.

For bruises and swelling (sprains and arthritis) make as strong a solution as you can tolerate: *We used kerosene cans* [laughs]. *We boiled up a whole bunch, and left it* [to cool]. *Then we soaked in it. For arthritis and swelling, you can put the can on a stove and keep it heated warm. We pulled out the wormwood before soaking. We didn't strain it...* Poultice bruises and swellings until the pain is re-lieved. Soak as many times a day as you can, re-warming the water each time. When soaking, use as warm a solution as you can stand.

When poulticing for skin cancer, replace the poultice two or three times a day. Keep the poultice on most of the time until the skin cancer is healed.

For yeast infection and poison oak, make as strong a solution as you can tolerate. Wash several times a day.

For diabetic feet, use mostly wormwood and only a little bit of Jimson weed. *When you soak your feet in Jimson weed, it's going to absorb into your skin, so you can't do it too long... We do it for about twenty minutes... If they have a lot of sores, we don't use that one. We just use plain wormwood. But if their skin's not broken, then we can use a lot of the Jimson weed...* When pain isn't present, the use of Jimson weed is unnecessary. One cannot oversoak in wormwood itself.

Apply salves periodically until healed.

When Josephine was growing up, and the family cows got their udders packed with milk, a wormwood poultice was applied overnight so they could release the milk. Wormwood was put in hot water to bring out its oils. The poultice was held in place by a sack with a drawstring.

During Josephine's childhood, lice were called greybacks. When someone with lice came to visit, after they left, Josephine's grandmother spread ashes from the family woodstove all around the stove area where everyone had been sitting. At school, kerosene was the preferred treatment for children who arrived with nits in their hair.

Wormwood grows on riverbars.

See also: coltsfoot, heal-all, Jimson weed, Johnny-jump-up, plantain, ribbed, sagebrush, old, and eucalyptus. For more about poison oak remedies, see also: dandelion, manzanita, mullein, plantain, ribbed and wide-leaf, soaproot, Solomon seal, walnut, black, and oatmeal and ocean water in the non-herbal cures section.

Yarrow

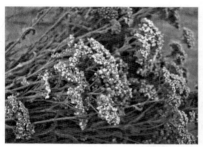

Dried yarrow. Photo by Beverly Ortiz.

LATIN NAME: *Achillea millefolium*

NATIVE PLANT: Yes

PART USED: Tops

USE: Fever and sore throat.

PREPARATION: Pick the flower heads, when they're starting to dry: *Everybody that picked it did it that way.* Hang upside down to complete the drying process. Store in a jar. To reduce fever, steep as a tea. To ease sore throat, make a warm gargle. For preparation details, see the section on gargles in "Types of Medicinals."

DOSAGE: Yarrow can be dangerous if consumed in large amounts. Use the standard ratio of one teaspoon to one cup of hot water for tea, but only drink a quarter of a cup at a time: *It's like taking the violet leaves. You start at a quarter of a cup...* If your fever doesn't start dropping with the first dose, you take another dose two hours later. Usually, two doses will break a fever, but take more if needed.

For a gargle for sore throat, steep at about the same strength as the tea, but make it stronger if a persistent cough exists. For dosage details, see the section on gargles in "Types of Medicinals."

The old people preferred yarrow for reducing fevers, but would use tansy if yarrow was unavailable.

See also: Johnny-jump-up and tansy.

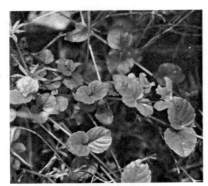

Yerba buena. Photo by Beverly Ortiz.

Yerba buena (vine tea, Indian tea)

KARUK NAME: champínnishich ["little-meadow-plant"]

LATIN NAME: *Satureja douglasii*

NATIVE PLANT: Yes

PART USED: Leaves and stem, including, when present, the flowers and the seeds that form underneath the leaves.

USE: Drink yerba buena tea, with its satisfying flavor, for pleasure. Use it to prevent and treat colds or flu, relieve fevers, and help firefighters' lungs. Also good for babies and young children with asthma and whooping cough. Use with yerba santa, heal-all, and Oregon grape root for cirrhosis of the liver or when the kidneys are giving out.

PREPARATION: Use fresh or dried. Steep as tea or make into a syrup.

For tea, steep a handful of the leaves and stem in a Pyrex pot filled with hot water. After steeping the tea for 20 minutes, it's unnecessary to remove the leaves.

For details on the preparation and use of syrups, see the section on syrups in "Types of Medicinals."

DOSAGE: To stop a cold or flu when you feel one coming on, or its associated fever, drink three cups of yerba buena tea, at as hot a temperature as you can handle, one right after the other. One such dose should be enough. If you don't take the tea after you get the cold or flu, it will reduce the symptoms rather than cure them. When taking the tea at this stage, drink two to three cups of yerba buena tea per day, spaced out throughout the day. Josephine makes yerba buena tea by the potful, then tries to finish it up in two days. Her children drink it up even faster: *You need to urinate a lot during the two days time to clear out your kidneys. They [the old people] used to say, "Flush them out." Then stop, since if you take it any longer, it will harm your kidneys.* Firefighters will brew up a five gallon container of yerba buena tea to help their lungs.

For babies and young children with asthma and whooping cough, make a cough syrup and give it to them twice daily, including once before bed—six millimeters out of a dropper for babies and one teaspoon for children. Give teenagers two teaspoons. Adults can take two teaspoons of syrup three to four times a day.

For cirrhosis of the liver, or when the kidneys are giving out, use about half a cup each of mountain balm, heal-all, Oregon grape root, and yerba buena to a gallon of water. Patients in the last stages of disease can drink it whenever they want.

When she finds them, Josephine tries to save yerba buena seeds to plant.

See also: angelica, heal-all, Oregon grape root, and mountain balm.

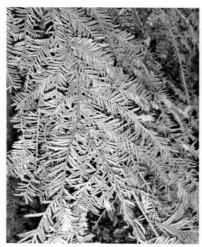

Yew. Photo by Frank Lake.

Yew

KARUK NAME: xuppáriish

LATIN NAME: *Taxus brevifolia*

NATIVE PLANT: Yes

PART USED: Inner bark.

USE: Any type of internal cancer.

PREPARATION: Gather the inner bark in the spring by pulling if away from the tree. Do not girdle the trees.

DOSAGE: Make the tea as strong as you can handle. Take one cup twice a day.

At one locale in Oregon, a dam flooded out and killed a yew forest.

CHAPTER FIVE

Non-Herbal Cures

Oatmeal

To relieve poison oak rash, add oatmeal to bath water or cook and press on face.

Ocean Water

To relieve poison oak rash, swim in ocean water.

Olive Oil

Rub olive oil on skin diseases, in particular psoriasis. Rub it, as well, for relief of arthritis. It's useful for healing radiation burns. In the latter case, carefully apply it to the unburned skin along the edge of the raw area.

Redmond Clay

Eat the clay to cleanse pinworms from the intestinal tract. "Were worms a problem when you were a kid?" I asked Josephine. *Sometimes*, she replied. *They were always saying, 'Don't eat this. Don't eat that. You'll get worms.' We weren't supposed to play in the mud or drink out of springs. We'd walk three miles when we went to school, and when it was hot, whenever we came to a spring along the road, we'd drink out of it... My dad used to try to keep the sediment cleaned out.*

Apply Redmond clay topically on insect bites and rashes. *This is the really bright looking red clay you see along the banks. We'd always get it and eat it. Everybody eats clay... If you're a potter, you'll eat clay. We used to get stung a lot, because we had beehives. We'd go irrigate, and with all the flowers in the alfalfa field [at the Old Home Place] we'd get stung. They'd pack that clay on it, and it stops the sting. It pulls that sting part out.*

Serpentine Mud

Give serpentine mud to patients with internal cancers and HIV/AIDS: *We go over and find a clean spring where the vegetation has rotted into it, and scoop it up, and eat the mud. A tablespoon of mud a day has enough arsenic in it to cure them.*

1. Over the years, basketweavers statewide have become increasing concerned about the effect of roadside herbicide spraying, since they commonly grip basketry materials with their teeth in order to split and debark them. Although it's more time-consuming to split and clean materials solely by hand, some weavers, fearing contamination, no longer use their teeth. While CalTrans has largely discontinued roadside spraying in Humboldt and Mendocino Counties, the California Indian Basketweavers Association continues to alert basketweavers to the potential problem.

2. Gargles may be made solely with salt.

3. An iodine solution may also be used for tonsillitis. Use about five drops in half a cup of water. With iodine, you have to rinse your mouth out with water when you get through. The mouth isn't rinsed when using seaweed or other gargles.

4. While it's more comfortable to use this rinse while warm, it can also be applied cold.

5. Josephine's grandmother used cold cream or other available jars, and Josephine still sometimes cleans out cold cream jars for the purpose.

6. The cows were milked into a bucket. From there the milk was strained through a cloth into a milk pan. The cream in the pan separated from the milk overnight. It was the children's job to skim off the cream with a spoon, then churn it. The family had a round, glass butter churn with wooden paddles. It was large enough to accommodate a pound to a pound and a half of butter. In wintertime the cream wouldn't sour for two or three days, but in the summer butter had to be churned everyday, a real chore for Josephine and her siblings. To keep the milk and butter fresh, the family had a screened-in "meat safe" in the shade outside their home. The safe was covered with burlap, its contents kept cool due to evaporation of cold water that was periodically poured over the burlap.

7. This recipe was provided by Zona Ferris and Jennifer Kalt, who joined Josephine in early spring with other project committee members who wanted to document and/or learn salve making—Bryan Colegrove, Patricia Ferris, LaVerne Glaze, Deborah McConnell, Kathy McCovey, and Quetta Peters. Although this meeting at the Hoopa Valley home of Deborah McConnell occurred on March 10, 2004, before the first full moon in April, and the plants, such as plantain, had relatively small leaves, Bryan, Kathy, and Virg McLaughlin located enough herbs of the proper size for the purpose. Since the wormwood wasn't yet tall enough, Josephine substituted dried wormwood flowers. Additional details were added to the recipe by Beverly Ortiz, as shared by Josephine Peters verbally.

8. Alternatively, a Pyrex pan may be used.

9. A screen strainer was used this day.

10. Alternatively, ½ pint canning jars may be used.

11. Alternatively, stir with a wooden spoon or Popsicle stick.

12. See endnote vii for context.

13. Coltsfoot is particularly useful for treating ulcerated and cancerous sores.

14. When using fresh wormwood, add it at the same time as the dried.

15. A screen strainer was used this day.

16. No woodstove was available this day.

17. This recipe came from Josephine verbally.

18. Josephine can obtain ribbed plantain year-round in her yard, although wide-leaved plantain dies down. Dandelion also dies down, and will only resprout after the first rains of spring, never when irrigated.

19. Excessive alcohol consumption can prevent sores from healing.

20. This recipe came from Josephine verbally. She generally uses peppernut meats to treat sores that don't heal. For large, open sores, like ulcerated sores on the legs, she generally makes a coltsfoot poultice.

21. Shake is comprised of the small leaves and partial pieces of bud trimmed off the big buds to make them more aesthetically pleasing. Less potent and less valued than what remains, shake is often used for things like making marijuana butter for baking. As a sort of by-product, shake isn't typically sold, but rather given away (Jennifer Kalt, personal communication, 9/19/04).

22. This recipe was recorded by Zona Ferris and Jennifer Kalt on March 10, 2004 (see endnote vii for details).

23. This recipe came from Josephine verbally.

24. Ibid.

25. When making "Indian bread" Josephine uses five cups of flour, about three-quarters of a cup of water, and, "nowadays," a pinch of salt. Put the dough in a greased pan, and pat it out flat, until it's about half an inch thick. Place in an oven preheated to 350°. Remove when browned. Eat as is.

26. Mary Ike from Somes Bar, Georgia Orcutt of Orleans, and interpreter Mamie Offield, also of Somes Bar.

27. Raleigh was a brand of medicines.

28. *xáap* is the Karuk name for thimbleberry, *Rubus parviflorus*.

29. The Karuk name for black (five-finger) fern and maidenhair fern is the same.

30. Tonic is synonymous with syrup.

31. Synonym *Brodiaea pulchella* (blue dicks).

32. Synonym *B. congestum*.

33. Synonym *B. multilflorum*.

34. Synonym *B. laxa*.

35. On private forest lands, foresters use herbicides to kill plants considered competitors to timber species, such as madrone, alder, ceanothus (soapbrush), manzanita, and tanoak, all species important to the Karuk. Sometimes foresters poison the whole plant, then bulldoze them down. Other times, they cut down the plant. All but ceanothus stump sprout, and are then sprayed to kill them. When removing bark from madrone stumps for medicinal purposes, care should be taken to insure the stumps don't occur on private timber lands, and haven't been sprayed (Jennifer Kalt, personal communication, 5/15/05).

36. Mormon tea was sometimes called squaw tea. According to Josephine, because of the connotations that have been placed on the word "squaw" in modern times, this has become a derogatory name. The same is true of yerba santa.

37. *uthkanpáhiip* is the Karuk name for coast redwood (*Sequoia sempervirens*).

Allen, Betty
    1957   Indians Teach Teachers. Northwestern California Roundup, The
               Humboldt Times July 6: p. 9.

Angulo, Jaime, and Lucy S. Freeland
    1931   Karok Texts. International Journal of American Linguistics
               6(3–4):194–226.

Arnold, Mary Ellicott, and Mabel Reed
    1957   In the Land of the Grasshopper Song: A Story of Two Girls in
               Indian Country in 1908–09. New York: Vantage Press.

Arthurs, Sara Watson
    2005   Local Students Get Science Fair Honors. Eureka Times-Standard,
               May 30 (Jennifer Kalt personal archive).

Baker, Marc Andre
    1981   The Ethnobotany of the Yurok, Tolowa, and Karok Indians of
               Northwest California. M.A. thesis, Humboldt State University, Arcata,
               CA.

Bell, Maureen
    1991   Karuk, the Upriver People. Happy Camp, CA: Naturegraph Publishers, Inc.
               Blue Lake Advocate.

    1966   Indians [sic] Pageant at Humboldt County Fair Brings Primitive
               Story: A Heritage Is Displayed, August 11 (Josephine Peters personal
               archive).

Bosworth, June
    1967   Nearly Lost Tradition of Basketry Being Returned by Hoopa Artisans.
               California-Oregon Roundup. Humboldt Times, April 4:11.

Bright, William
    1954   The Travels of Coyote, a Karok Myth. Kroeber Anthropological Society
               Papers 11:1–17. Berkeley: University of California.
    1957   The Karok Language. University of California Publications in
               Linguistics 13. Berkeley: University of California.
    1978   Karok. In Handbook of North American Indians, Volume 8, California,
               Robert F. Heizer, ed. Pp. 180–189. Washington, DC: Smithsonian
               Institution.

Buckley, Thomas
    2002   Standing Ground, Yurok Indian Spirituality 1850–1990. Berkeley:
               University of California Press.

Cohodas, Marvin
    1997   Basketweavers for the California Curio Trade: Elizabeth and Louise
               Hitckox. Tucson: University of Arizona Press, and Los Angeles:
               Southwest Museum.

Colegrove, Bryan
>   2004   Personal communication with Jennifer Kalt.

Common Sense
>   1980   Lorencita Masten, August 4:8, 11.
>   1980a   Holistic Medicine, August 1810.
>   1980b   Indian Doctor Visits, November 24:14.
>   1980c   Hoopa Medical Center: The History, the Beginning, and the Man Behind the Dream, December 8:10–12.

Davis, Barbara J., and Michael Hendryx
>   1991   Plants and the People: The Ethnototany of the Karuk Tribe. Yreka, CA: Siskiyou County Museum.

Emery, Dara
>   1988   Seed Propagation of Native California Plants. Santa Barbara, CA: Santa Barbara Botanic Garden.

Ferndale Enterprise
>   1966   Indian Customs, Native Culture Return to Fair, August 18:1, 4.

Ferrara, James
>   n.d   Plant and Animal Names Composite List with English Glosses of Karuk Terms. Orleans: Karuk Tribe of California.
>   2004   Scientific (Latin) Designations for Plants, with Corresponding Karuk Names. Draft 4, March 8. Orleans: Karuk Tribe of California.

Gendron, Hazel Davis, and Beck, Cheryl M.
>   2009   Gold Rush and the Mixing of Cultures in Western Siskiyou County. Siskiyou Pioneer 8(9):7-51.

Grant III, Frank A.
>   1972   The Grant Family. Siskiyou Pioneer 4(2):15–20.
>   2000   Documentation of Francis Brazille (1827–1878) as Indian. Manuscript in possession of author.

Graves, Charles Sumner
>   1929   Lore and Legends of the Klamath River Indians. Yreka, CA: Press of the Times.
>   1934   Before the White Man Came. Yreka, CA: The Siskiyou News.

Harrington, John Peabody
>   1931   Karuk Texts. International Journal of American Linguistics 107.
>   1932a   Karuk Indian Myths. Bureau of American Ethnology Bulletin 107: 1–34.
>   1932b   Tobacco among the Karuk Indians of California. Bureau of American Ethnology Bulletin 94:1–47.

Heffner, Kathy
>   1984   "Following the Smoke": Contemporary Plant Procurement by the Indians of Northwest California. Eureka, CA: Six Rivers National Forest.

Heizer, Robert F., ed.
>   1967   Ethnological Notes on Northern and Southern California Indian Tribes. University of California Archaeological Reports 68, Part 2.

Hickman, James C., ed.
>   1993   The Jepson Manual: Higher Plants of California. Berkeley and Los Angeles: University of California Press.

Hotelling, Wesley E.
1978   My Life with the Kar-ooks, Miners and Forestry. Self published, Willow Creek, CA.

Jepson Manual On-Line, The
2008   Index to Treatment and Keys from The Jepson Manual. Jepson Flora Project: Jepson Interchange. http://ucjeps.berkeley.edu/interchange/I_treat_indexes.html.

Johnson, Ron, and Coleen Kelley Marks
1997   Her Mind Made Up: Weaving Caps the Indian Way. Arcata, CA: Humboldt State University.

Kellems, Ann
1970   Indian Arts now Offered in Hoopa. Unidentified newspaper, December 30. Original in scrapbook in possession of Josephine Peters.

Kelly, Isabel T.
1930   The Carver's Art of the Indians of Northwestern California. University of California Publications in American Archaeology and Ethnology 24(7):103–119.

Kelsey, Andrea, ed.
1981   Common Sense, December 7:6.

Klam-ity Kourier
1968   Indian Artistry Is Not Dead, January 17:7.
1969   Rock Shop Museum Holds Many Treasures, November 19:8.

Kroeber, Alfred, A. L., and E. W. Gifford
1980   Karok Myths. Grace Buzaljko, ed. Berkeley: University of California Press.

Lake, Frank K.
2007   "Traditional Ecological Knowledge to Develop and Maintain Fire Regimes in Northwestern California, Klamath-Siskiyou Bioregion: Management and Restoration of Culturally Significant Habitats". Ph.D. dissertation, Environmental Sciences, Oregon State University.

Lang, Julian
1994   Ararapíkva, Creation Stories of the People: Traditional Karuk Indian Literature from Northwestern California. Berkeley, CA: Heyday Books.

LaPena, Frank
1987   Reflections of a Changing Earth. News from Native California 1(1):14. Marshall, Rain, interviewer.
1999   Northwest Indigenous Gold Rush History: The Indian Survivors of California's Holocaust. Chag Lowry, ed. Indian Teacher and Educational Personnel Program. Eureka, CA: Humboldt State University.
Mills, Elaine L., ed.

1985   The Papers of John Peabody Harrington in the Smithsonian Institution, 1907–1957, Volume 2, A Guide to the Field Notes, Native American History, Language and Culture of Northern and Central California. White Plains, NY: Kraus International Publications.

Most, Stephen
2006   River of Renewal: Myth and History in the Klamath Basin. Portland: Oregon Historical Society Press in association with University of Washington Press.

Navarro, Linda D.

2000/01 The Committee for Traditional Indian Health: A Program of the California Rural Indian Health Board. News from Native California 14(2):22–24.

Ortiz, Beverly R.

1988   Baskets of Dreams. News from Native California 2(4):28–29.

1989   Mount Diablo as Myth and Reality: An Indian History Convoluted. The American Indian Quarterly 13(4):457–470.

1998   Following the Smoke: Karuk Indigenous Basketweavers and the Forest Service. News from Native California 11(3):21–29.

1999   Following the Smoke II: Plants and the Karuk. News from Native California 12(3):13–16.

1999/00 "In Those Days We Had a Lot of Time": Iris Fiber Cordage. News from Native California 13(2):29–33.

2002   Eating Poison Oak: Alex Ramirez's Childhood. A Gathering of Voices: The Native Peoples of the Central California Coast. Linda Yamane, ed. Santa Cruz County History Journal 5:157–160.

Peters, Josephine

1950s–70s Scrapbook of articles from the 1950s through 1970s, most undated. The articles were compiled from the Blue Lake Advocate, Del Norte Triplicate, Ferndale Enterprise, Humboldt Times, Klam-ity Kourier, Medford Mail Tribune, Record-Searchlight (Redding), The Sacramento Bee, Siskiyou Daily News, and Times-Standard (Eureka), all California. Scrapbook in possession of Josephine Peters.

Pilling, Arnold

1978   Yurok. Handbook of North American Indians, Volume 8, California, Robert F. Heizer, ed. Pp. 137–154. Washington, DC: Smithsonian Institution.

Reese Bullen Gallery

1991   Elizabeth Conrad Hickox, Baskets from the Center of the World. Eureka, CA: Humboldt State University.

Roberts, Linda, et al.

1999   Cultural Plants and Healing List. A Guide to Plants and Cultural Recipes Used by Northwest California Indians. Sumeg/Patrick's Point/ Lagoon Interpretive Association.

Rose, Robin, Caryn E. C. Chachulski, and Diane L. Haase

1998   Propagation of Pacific Northwest Native Plants. Corvallis: Oregon State University Press.

Sanderson, Grover C. [Eaglewing, Chief]

2001   [1938] Peek-Wa Stories: Ancient Indian Legends of California. Santa Clara, CA: DeHart's Printing Services.

Schenck, Sara M., and E. W. Gifford

1952   Karok Ethnobotany. Anthropological Records 13(6):397–392.

Sharp, Nelson

1966   Ancient Art of Basket Weaving Being Revived Through Hoopa Classes. Unidentified newspaper. Original in scrapbook in possession of Josephine Peters.

Silver, Shirley
    1978   Shastan Peoples. Handbook of North American Indians, Volume 8,
            California, Robert F. Heizer, ed. Pp. 211–224. Washington, DC:
            Smithsonian Institution.

Small, Mark
    1980   Introducing: Hoopa Valley's Traditional Medicine Program. Common
            Sense, Early June:10.

Tilford, Gregory L.
    1998   From Earth to Herbalist. Missoula, MT: Mountain Press Publishing.

Wallace, William J.
    1978   Hupa, Chilula, and Wilkut. Handbook of North American Indians,
            Volume 8, California, Robert F. Heizer, ed. Pp. 137–154. Washington,
            DC: Smithsonian Institution.

Wistar, Issac J.
    1937   [1914] Autobiography of Issac Jones Wistar 1827–1905. Philadelphia:
            The Wistar Institute of Anatomy and Biology.

Note: boldface page numbers in this index indicate detailed plant descriptions.

Acer macrophyllum, 104
Achillea millefolium, 194
achnat'apvuytiiv, 166
achnatsinvánnahich, 170
achnatsinvannahíchkaam, 170
Achyls californica, 187
Adiantum aleuticum, 123
Adiantum jordanii, 124
Agaricus bisporus, 154
akviin, 155
akvíttip, 101
alder, 28, 200
alder, red, 101
alder, white, **101**, 183
alfalfa, **101–102**, 134, 197
Allium acuminatum, 158
    A. amplectens, 158
    A. bolanderi, 158
    A. campanulatum, 158
    A. cratericola, 158
    A. falcifolium, 158
    A. hoffmanii, 158
    A. membranaceum, 158
    A. paniculatum var. *paniculatum*,
      158
    A. siskiyouense, 158
    A. unifolium, 158
    A. validum, 158
    A. vineale, 158
Allium sativum, 126
Alnus rhombifolia, 101
Alnus rubra, 101
Amthemis arvensis, 165
anach'úhish, 150
angelica, *see* Indian root
Angelica sinensis, 121
Angelica tomentosa, 138
annúphiich, 151
Anthemis cotula, 106
apple, domestic, 42, 78, 91, 92, 97, **102**
apxantich'athithxuntapan'íppa(ha),189
Aralia californica, 181
Arbutus menziesii, 147
Arctostaphylos canescens, 148
    A. canescens subsp. *sonomensis*,148
    A. columbiana, 148
    A. glandulosa, 148
    A. hispidula, 148

A. klamathensis, 148
A. manzanita, 148
A. nevadensis, 148
A. nortensis, 148
A. patula, 148
A. viscida, 148
A. viscida subsp. *pulchella*, 148
A. viscida subsp. *viscida*, 148
Armillaria ponderosa, 154
Artemesia douglasiana, 192
Artemisia ludoviciana subsp. *lu
    doviciana*, 192
Artemesia tridentata, 171
artichoke, **102**
artichoke, Jerusalem, **103**, 117
asáppiip, 115
Asarum hartwegii, 127
Asclepias eriocarpa, 149
Asclepias tuberosa, 167
attaychúrip, 104
axmúhishanach ichxúunanach, 112
axráttip, 130
axvêep, 156, 157
axyússip, 164
banana, **103**
barberry, **103–104**
bay, *see* peppernut
bay laurel, *see* peppernut
bear berry, *see* spikenard
Berberis aquifolium, 103, 104
Berberis nervosa, 158
Berberis vulgaris, 104
berry, Christmas, *see* toyon
berry, Himalaya, *see* Himalaya berry
big-leaf maple, 94, **104**, 138
blackberry, California, *see* blackberry,
    wild
blackberry, wild, 89, 92, 145, **104**
blackcap, 89, 91, 92, **105**
black cohosh, *see* cohosh, black
black cottonwood, *see* cottonwood,
    black
black fern, *see* fern, black
black jack, **106**, 145
black oak, *see* oak
black walnut, *see* walnut, black
blood root, **106**, 162, 173, 180
blue camas, *see* Indian potato

blue cohosh, *see* cohosh, blue
blue elderberry, *see* elderberry, blue
Brassica rapa, 154
    B. nigra, 154
Brodiaea coronaria, 138
    B. elegans, 138
buckbrush, *see* greasewood
burdock, 77, **107**
California blackberry, *see* blackberry,
    wild
California ginseng, *see* ginseng,
    California
California licorice, *see* black jack
California rose, *see* rose, California
Calocedrus decurrens, 137
Calypso bulbosa, 142
Cantherellus cibarius, 154
canyon live oak, *see* oak
Capsella bursa-pastoris, 175
capsicum, *see* cayenne
caraway, wild, **107**
cardinal flower, *see* lobelia, cardinal
Carthamus tinctorius, 171
cascara, *see* chitem bark
cascara buckthorn, *see* chitem bark
catnip, **108**, 127
Caulophyllum thalictroides, 114
cayenne (hot pepper), **108**, 146
ceanothus, *see* soapbrush
Ceanothus integerrimus, 177
Ceanothus velutinus, 131
cedar, 51, *see also* cedar, incense
cedar, incense, *see* incense cedar
cedar, Port Orford, *see* Port Orford cedar
Centella asiatica, 130
chamomile, *see* pineapple plant
Chamomilla recutita, 165
    C. occidentalis, 165
    C. suaveolens, 165
champínnishich, 195
chantínnihiich, 175
chantiripirishpírishhitihan, 120
chantrelle mushrooms, *see* mushrooms,
    chantrelle
chaparral, *see* sagebrush, old
cheeseweed, **109**
cherry, 28
cherry, wild, *see* choke-cherry, wild

chickweed, 72, 77, **110**, 150, 169
chicory, **110**
Chimaphila umbellata, 165
chitem bark, **111**
Chloragalum pomeridianum, 178
choke-cherry, wild (wild cherry), 73,
74, 75, 81, 88, **111–112**, 120,
121, 133, 150, 152
Christmas berry, *see* toyon
chuneexneeyâach, 137
cicely, sweet, *see* black jack
Cichorum intybus, 110
citronella, *see* lemon mint
Claytonia perfoliata subsp. *perfoliata*,
150
clover, elk, *see* ginseng, California
clover, pink, 77, **112**
clover, red, *see* clover, pink
clover, white, 81, **113**, 118, 166
cluster rose, *see* rose, cluster
coast tea, *see* swamp tea
cocklebur, *see* burdock
cohosh, black, **114**
cohosh, blue, **114**
coltsfoot, 50, 84, 85, 86, 94, **114–115**,
133, 140, 166, 193, 199, 200
commercial ginger, *see* ginger,
commercial
commercial ginseng, *see* ginseng,
commercial
commercial mushrooms, *see*
mushrooms, commercial
commercial sage, *see* sage, commercial
Commiphora myrrha, 155
corn, **115**
Cornus nuttallii, 120
Corylus cornuta var. *californica*, 133
cottonwood, 86, **115**, 153, 166, 177
cottonwood, black, *see* cottonwood
coyote mint, *see* pennyroyal
cranesbill, **116**
Crataegus oxyacanthus, 132
C. douglasii, 132
C. mouogyna , 132
cucumber, 98, **116**
Cucumis sativus, 116
curly dock, *see* dock, curly
currant, domestic, **116**
currant, red flowering, 72, **116**, 156
Cymbopogon hirtus, 143
C. citrates, 143
C. flexuous, 143
Cynara scolymus, 102
Cypripedium californicum, 142
dahlia, **117**
Dahlia spp., 117

damiana, **117–118**
dandelion, 84, 86, 113, **118–119**, 149,
153, 166, 200
Darmera peltata, 145
Datura wrightii, 140
D. stramonium, 140
deer oak, *see* oak
devil's club, 50, 77, **119**
Dichelostemma capitatum, 138
D. congestum, 138
D. multilflorum, 138
Dichelostemma ida-maia, 125
Disporum sp., 178
D. smithii, 178
dock, curly, 77, 129, **120**
dock, yellow, *see* dock, curly
dog fennel, 106
dog rose, *see* rose, dog
dogwood, 74, 75, 111, 112, **120–121**,150
domestic currant, *see* currant, domestic
domestic peach, *see* peach, domestic
domestic red raspberry, **105**
dong quai, **121**
Douglas fir, *see* fir, Douglas
Durango root, 28
dwarf trillium, *see* motherwort
Eastern tobacco, *see* tobacco, Eastern
echinacea, 76, 77, **121**
Echinacea purpurea, 121
E. angustifolia, 121
E. pallida, 121
elderberry, blue, **122**
elk clover, *see* ginseng, California
Ephedra sp., 151
E. nevadensis, 151
E. viridis, 151
Equisetum telmateia subsp. *braunii*,
188
Eriodictyon californicum, 152
Erodium botrys, 116
E. brachycarpum, 116
E. cicutarium, 116
E. moschatum, 116
Erysimum capitatum var. *capitatum*,
188
eucalyptus, **122**
Eucalyptus spp., 122
Euphrasia offinale, 122
E. rostkoviana, 122
eyebright, **122–123**
false hellebore, *see* hellebore, false
false Solomon's seal, *see* Solomon seal
fáththip, 148
fath'uruhsa'ippa, 148
fat Solomon seal, *see* Solomon seal
fenugreek, **123**

fern, black, 28, 78, **123**, 200
fern, five-finger, *see* fern, black
fern, licorice, *see* licorice fern
fern, maidenhair, **124**
Ficus carica, 124
fig, 41, **124**
filaree, *see* cranesbill
fir, *see* fir, white
fir, Douglas, 28, 30, 75, **125**
fir, white, 51, 170
firecracker Flower, **125**
five-finger fern, *see* fern, black
Foeniculum vulgaris, 144
foxglove, 111, 120
Fragaria vesca, 182
garden violet, 115, **140–141**, 166, 193
garlic, 41, 98, **126**, 159
Gaultheria shallon, 172
geranium (commercial), 73,116,**126–127**
geranium, wild, 73, 116
germander, *see* cranesbill
ginger, commercial, 73, **127**, 171, 172
ginger, white, 51, 73, 108, **127**, 136, 171
ginseng family, 181
ginseng, California, 13, 105, **128**, 136
ginseng, commercial, 105, **128**, 136
ginseng, white, *see* California ginseng
goldenseal, 76–77, 80, **129**, 162, 180,
189
Goodyera oblongifolia, 166
gooseberry, 90, **130**, 149, 188
gotu kola, 74, **130**
grape, Oregon, *see* Oregon grape
grape, wild, 19, 72, **131**
gray pine, *see* pine
gray willow, *see* willow, gray
greasewood, **131**
greenleaf manzanita, *see* manzanita,
greenleaf
grindelia, 71, 72, 73, 75, 80, 123, 129,
132, 156, 160, 161–162
Grindelia hirsutula, 132
ground rose, *see* rose, ground
gum plant, *see* grindelia
hawthorn, **132**
hazel, 12, 28, 56, 43, 58, **133**, 189, 192
heal-all, 76, 77, 85, 88, 111, 115,
133–134, 140, 150, 152, 158,
159, 193, 195
Helianthus tuberosus, 103
hellebore, false, **134**
Heteromeles arbutifolia, 186
Himalaya berry, 91, **104**
hops, **134–135**
horehound, 86, 87, 88, 89, **135**, 152
horsetail, *see* wahoo

ho shou wu, **136**

hot pepper, *see* cayenne

huckleberry, 28, 31, 118, **137**

huckleberry oak, *see* oak

Humulus lupulus, 134

Hydrastis Canadensis, 129

Hypericum perforatum, 182

ihêeraha, 185

ihyivkâanvar, 158

ikrittápkir yumareekrittápkir, 123, 124

ikshassahánnihich iíftihan, 151imkanva'u xpirishpírishhitihan, 106

imyúha, 178

incense cedar, **137**, 150

Indian potato, **138**, 158

Indian rhubarb, *see* lily, pond

Indian root, 28, 72, 77, 106, 107, **138–139**

Indian tea, *see* Mormon tea and yerba buena

Indian tobacco, *see* tobacco, Indian

iris, 30, **139**

Irish moss, 174, *see* seaweed

Iris macrosiphon, 139

ishmúchchah, 173

ishvakíppish, 164

ishvírip, 164

itháriip, 125

(i)thivthaneentáayvar pinishxanahyâachas, 182

Jeffrey pine, *see* pine

Jerusalem artichoke, *see* artichoke, Jerusalem

jimson weed, 132, **140**, 193–194

Johnny-jump-up, 73, 84–85, 86, 115, 122, 133, **140–141**, 167, 193, 194

joint weed, *see* lady's thumb

Juglans californica var. *hindsii*, 189

juniper, **141–142**

Juniperus communis, 141

   J. occidentalis, 141

   J. osteasperma, 141

káaf, 145

káat, 192

kíthriip, 177

Klamath plum, *see* plum Klamath

Klamath weed, *see* St. John's wort

knotweed, 48, **142**, 143

kuríthxiit, 138

kusríppan, 147

kusríppish, 147

kusvêep, 168

Labrador tea, 75, 76, 127, *see* swamp tea

lady slipper, pink, 48, 76, **142**, 150

lady slipper, white, 48, 76, **142**, 150,

162, 176

lady's thumb, **143**

laurel, bay, *see* peppernut

laurel, mountain, *see* soapbrush

Ledum glandulosum, 183

lemon grass, **143**

lemon mint, 78, 127, **144**

licorice, California, *see* black jack

licorice fern, **144**

licorice plant (licorice), **144**, 146

licorice root, **145**

Ligusticum californicum, 107

   L. grayi, 107

lily, pond, 104, **145**

lily, skunk, *see* skunk lily

Lithocarpus densiflorus, 183

lobelia, blue, 72, 108, **146**, 176

lobelia, cardinal, 72, **146**

Lobelia inflata, 146

lobelia, red, *see* lobelia, cardinal

Lysichiton americanum, 176

madrone, 30, 138, **147**, 200

mahímkaanva, 138

mallow, *see* cheeseweed

Malus, 102

Malva parviflora, 109

maple, *see* big-leaf maple

manzanita, 65, 90, **148–149**, 200

manzanita, greenleaf, 148

manzanita, Parry, 148

Marrubium vulgare, 135

maul oak, *see* oak

Medicago sativa, 101

Melissa officinalis, 144

Mentha piperita, 162

Mentha spicata var. *spicata*, 180

milk thistle, *see* thistle, milk

milkweed, 60, 72, **149**, 167

Mimulus cardinalis, 146

Mimulus guttatus, 151

miner's lettuce, 77, 110, **150**, 169

mistletoe, 76, 142, 150, 162, 176

mitimshaxvuh'íppa, 149

Monardella odoratissima, 161

monkeyflower, yellow, **151**

Mormon tea, 76, 77, **151**, 200

motherwort (dwarf trillium, trillium), 13, **151**

mountain balm (yerba santa), 72, 74, 75, 86, 87, 88, 89, 90, 94, 109, 111, 130, 133, 135, **152**, 158, 159, 172, 195, 200

mountain laurel, *see* soapbrush

mugwort, *see* wormwood

múhish, 106

mullein, *see* mullein, wild

mullein, wild, 118, **152–153**

Musa, 103

mushrooms, chanterelle, 28, 69, 73, 93, 127, 147, **154**

mushrooms, commercial, 73, 93, 147, **154**

mushrooms, tanoak, 28, 69, 73, 93, 127, 147, **154**

mustard, yellow, 81, **154**

myrrh, **155**, 177

myrtlewood, *see* peppernut

neevxâat, 155

Nepeta cataria, 108

nettle, **155**

Nicotiana sp., 185

   N. tabacum, 185

Nicotiana quadrivalvis, 185

   N. bigelovii, 185

ninebark, **156**

Nootka rose, *see* rose, Nootka

oak, 30, 42, 94, 95, 144, 150, **156–157**, 170, *see also* mushrooms, tanoak, oak, white and valley, and tanoak

oak, black, 156, *see* oak

oak, canyon live, 156, *see* oak

oak, deer, 156, *see* oak

oak, huckleberry, 156, *see* oak

oak, maul, 156, *see* oak

oak, mistletoe, 150

oak, Oregon, 156, 157, *see* oak, and oak, white

oak, poison, *see* poison oak

oak, white, 94, 95, 156, **157**, 170, *see also* oak

oak, valley, 95, *see also* oak

Oemleria cerasiformis, 160

old man's beard, *see* reindeer moss

old sagebrush, *see* sagebrush, old

onion, wild, **158**

Oplopanax horridus, 119

Oregon grape, 107, 120, **158–159**

Oregon grape, tall, *see* barberry

Oregon oak, *see* oak

Osmorhiza berteroi, 106

   O. chilensis, 106

Osmorhiza occidentalis, 106, 107

oso berry, *see* peach, wild

Oxalis oregana, 179

pâarak, 190

pahav'íppa, 148

pahiip, 162

Panax quinqufolius, 128

Parry manzanita, *see* manzanita, Parry

parsley, **159**

Passiflora spp., 160

passion flower, **160**
pasyiip, 186
paturúpveen'ippa(ha), 105
peach, domestic, 73, 76, 78, 91, 92, 97, 121 **160**, 182, 183
peach, wild, 121, 132, 156, **160–161**
Pelargonium spp., 126
pennyroyal, 75, **161–162**
Penstemon sp., 176
    P. anguineus, 176
    P. azureus, 176
    P. azureus var. *azureus*, 176
    P. davidsonii var *davidsonii*, 176
    P. deustus, 176
    P. deustus var. *suffrutescens*, 176
    P. filifornis, 176
    P. heterodoxus, 176
    P. heterodoxus var. *heterodoxus*, 176
    P. heterophuyllus, 176
    P. heterophyllus var. *heterophyllus*, 176
    P. laetus, 176
    P. laetus var. *sagittatus*, 176
    P. newberryi, 176
    P. newberryi var. *berryi*, 176
    P. parvulus, 176
    P. procerus, 176
    P. procerus var. *brachyanthus*, 176
    P. procerus var. *formosus*, 176
    P. purpusii, 176
    P. rattanii, 176
    P. rattanii var. *rattanii*, 176
    P. roezlii, 176
    P. rupicola, 176
    P. speciosus, 176
    P. tracyi, 176
pepper, hot, 98, *see* cayenne
peppermint, 75, 78, 106, 127, 129, **162**, 191
peppernut, 23, 25, 28, 42, 50, 77, 78, 81, 86, 95–96, 134, 153, **162–164**, 190, 200
Petasites frigidus var. *palmatus*, 114
Petroselinum crispum, 159
Phoradendron villosum, 150
    P. densum, 150
    P. libocedri, 150
    P. villosum, 150
Physocarpus capitatus, 156
pihneefyukkúkkuh, 142
pikvassáhiich, 178
pine, 28, 30, **164**, *see also* pine nut beads, pine nuts, and pine pitch
pine, gray, 30, 56, 96, 164
pine, Jeffrey, 164, *see* pine
pine, piñon, 96

pine, ponderosa, 164, *see* pine
pine, sugar, 164, *see* pine
pineapple plant (chamomile), 71, 160, **165**
pineapple weed, *see* pineapple plant
piñon pine, *see* pine, piñon
Pinus spp., 164
    P. albicoulis, 164
    P. attentuata, 164
    P. balfouriana, 164
    P. balfouriana subsp. *boufouriana*, 164
    P. contorta, 164
    P. contorta subsp. *murrayana*, 164
    P. jeffreyi, 164
    P. lambertiana, 164
    P. monticola, 164
    P. ponderosa, 164
    P. sabiniana, 164
pink clover, *see* clover, pink
pink lady slipper, *see* lady slipper, pink
pipsissewa, **165**, 191
pirish'axvâaharas, 152
Plantago lanceolata, 166
Plantago major, 166
Plantago psyllium, 168
plantain (for baskets), 43, *see* plantain, ribbed
plantain, narrow, *see* plantain, ribbed
plantain, rattlesnake, **166**
plantain, ribbed (narrow), 84, 86, 113, 115, 118, 119, 140, 153, **166–167**, 178, 193, 199, 200
plantain, wide-leaf, 84, 86, 113, 115, 118, 119, 140, 153, **166–167**, 178, 193, 199, 200
pleurisy root, **167**
plum, Klamath, **167**
poison oak, 79, 80, 81, 84, 118, 148, 153, 166, **168**, 178, 179, 189, 192, 193, 197
Polygonum arenastrum, 142
Polygonum multifloum, 136
Polygonum persicaria, 143
Polypodium glyccyrhiza, 144
Ponderosa pine, *see* pine
pond lily, *see* lily, pond
Populus balsamifera subsp. *trichocarpa*, 115
Port Orford cedar, 68
Portulaca oleracea, 169
potato, Indian, *see* Indian potato
prince's pine, *see* pipsissewa
princess pine, *see* pipsissewa
Prunella vulgaris, 133
Prunus persica, 160
Prunus subcordata, 167

Prunus virginiana var. *demissa*, p. 111
Pseudotsuga menziesii, 125
psyllium, **168–169**
pufichxannáchyuh, 158
puke root, *see* dock, curly
pulsane, *see* purslane
purith'íppan, 137
purithkam'ippa(ha), 172
purslane, **169–170**, 180
púun, 111
Pyrola picta, 191
Quercus spp., 156
    Q. chrysolepis, 156
    Q. garryana, 156
    Q. garryana var. *brewerii*, 156
    Q. garryana var. *garryana*, 156
    Q. kelloggii, 156
    Q. sadleriana, 156
    Q. vacciniifolia, 156
Quercus garryana, 157
raspberry, domestic red, *see* domestic red raspberry
raspberry, wild, *see* blackcap
rattlesnake plantain, *see* plantain, rattlesnake
red alder, *see* alder, red
red clover, *see* clover, pink
red flowering currant, *see* currant, red flowering
red lobelia, *see* lobelia cardinal
red raspberry, domestic, *see* blackcap
redwood sorrel, *see* sorrel, redwood
reindeer moss, **170**
Rhamnus purshiana, 111
Rhus diversiloba, 168
ribbed plantain, *see* plantain, ribbed
Ribes nigrum, 117
Ribes roezlii var. *cruentum*, 130
Ribes sanguineum var. *sanguineum*, 117
Rorippa nasturtium–aquaticum, 190
Rosa spp., 170
    R. californica, 170
    R. canina, 170
    R. eglanteria, 170
    R. gymnocarpa, 170
    R. nutkana var. *nutkana*, 170
    R. pisocarpa, 170
    R. spithamea, 170
rose, California, **170**
rose, dog, **170**
rose, cluster, **170**
rose, ground, **170**
rose hips, **170–171**
rose, Nootka, 170
rose, wood, 170

Rubus discolor, 104
Rubus idaeus, 105
Rubus leucodermis, 105
Rubus parviflorus, 184
Rubus spectabilis, 173
Rubus ursinus, 104
Rumex acetosella, 180
Rumex crispus, 120
sáan, 104
safflower, **171**
sage, **171–172**
sagebrush, 152, 171–172
sagebrush, old, **172**, 193
sage, commercial, 171–172
sage, from down south, 171–172
sage, white, *see* sage from down south
salal, **172**
Salix exigua, 190
    S. hindsiana, 190
salmonberry, **173**
Salvia apiana, 171
Salvia officinalis, 171
Sambucus mexicana, 122
Sanguinaria canadensis, 106
sanicle, purple, **173**
Sanicula bipinnatifida, 173
sarsaparilla, **173–174**
sassafras, **174**
Sassifras albidum, 174
Satureja douglasii, 195
Scoliopus bigelovii, 184
Scutellaria antirhinnoides, 146, 176
seaweed, 28, 78, 96–97, 105, **174–175**, 199
self heal, *see* heal–all
sheep sorrel, *see* sourgrass
sheep's sorrel, *see* sourgrass
shepherd's purse, 108, **175**
Silybum marianum, 185
skullcap, 72, 76, **176**
skunk cabbage, **176**
skunk lily, *see* TB flower
slippery elm, 115, 155, **177**
Smilacina stellata, 178
    S. racemosa, 178
S. racemosa var. *amplexicaulis*, 178
Smilax officinalis, 173
soapbrush (ceanothus), 28, **177**, 200
soap plant, *see* soaproot
soaproot, **178**
Solomon seal, 48, 133, 134, 178, **178–179**
Solomon seal, fat, *see* Solomon seal
Solomon's seal, false, 178–179, *see* Solomon seal
Solomon's seal, fat, 178–179,

see Solomon seal
Solomon's seal, starry, *see* Solomon seal
sorrel, redwood, 28, 65, **179**
sourgrass, 118, **180**
spearmint, 75, 78, 106, 127, 129, 180–**181**
spikenard, 80, 81, 128, 178, **181**
starry Solomon's seal, *see* Solomon seal
star thistle, *see* thistle, star
St. James weed, *see* shepherd's purse
St. John's wort, 28, 48, 71, 72, 74, **182**
Stellaria media, 110
storksbill, *see* cranesbill
strawberry, wild, 105, **182**
string iris, *see* iris
sugar pine, *see* pine
sunchoke, *see* Artichoke, Jerusalem
sunroot, *see* Artichoke, Jerusalem
swamp tea (Labrador tea), 75, 76, 127, **183**
sweet-briar, 170
sweet cicely, *see* black jack
sweet fennel, *see* licorice plant
takkánnaafích, 179
tall Oregon grape, *see* barberry
Tanacetum camphoratum, 184
tanoak, 30, 93, 94, 101, 165 **183**, 200, *see also* mushrooms, tanoak
tanoak mushrooms, *see* mushrooms, tanoak
tansy, **184**, 194
tapasxávish, 156
Taraxacum officinale, 118
Taxus brevifolia, 196
TB flower, **184**
thámkaat, 161
thimbleberry, 119, **184**, 200
thistle, milk, **185**
thistle, star, 79, 114, **185**
thuf'áhan, 117
thukinpírish, 103, 158
tobacco, Eastern, **185**
tobacco, Indian, 72, 146, **185–186**, *see also* barberry and mountain balm
topinambur, *see* artichoke, Jerusalem
Toxicodendron diversilobum, 168
toyon, **186**
Tricholoma magnivelare, 154
Trifolium pratense, 112
T. arvense, 112
T. campestre, 112
T. glomeratum, 112
T. hirtum, 112
T. hybridum, 112
T. incarnatum, 112

T. pratense, 112
T. repens, 112
Trifolium repens, 113
    T. cyanthiferum, 113
    T. eriocephalum, 113
Trigonella foenum–graecum, 123
trillium, dwarf, *see* motherwort
Trillium ovatum subsp. *ovatum*, 151
    T. ovatum, 151
Triteleia bridgesii, 138
    T. laxa, 138
Tumera diffusa, 117
    T. diffusa var. *aphrodisiaca*, 117
Ulmus fulva, 177
Umbellularia californica, 162
Urtica dioica subsp. *gracilis*, 155
    U. californica, 155
    U. dioica subsp. *holosericea*, 155
    U. holosericea, 155
Usnea spp., 170
ússip, 164
uyáhaama, 120
uyhúrurip, 131
Vaccinium ovatum, 137
valerian, **186**
Valeriana sitchensis, 186
vanilla plant, **187**
Veratrum viride, 134
Verbascum thapsus, 152
Verbena lasiostachys, 187
vervain, **187**
vine tea, *see* yerba buena
Viola ocellata, 140
Viola sp., 140
    V. odorata, 140
violet, *see* Johnny jump–up
violet, garden, *see* garden violet
Vitus californicus
wahoo, **188**
wallflower, **188**
walnut, black, 95, 105, 109, **189**
watercress, **190**
white alder, *see* alder, white
white clover, *see* clover, white
white fir, *see* fir, white
white ginger, *see* ginger, white
white ginseng, *see* California ginseng
white lady slipper, *see* lady slipper, white
white oak, *see* oak, white
white sage, *see* sage from down south
white-veined wild ginger, *see* ginger, white
wide-leaf plantain, *see* plantain, wide-leaf
wild caraway, *see* caraway, wild

wild cherry, *see* choke-cherry, wild
wild choke-cherry, *see* choke-cherry,
   wild
wild geranium, *see* geranium, wild
wild ginger, *see* ginger, white
wild mullein, *see* mullein, wild
wild onion, *see* onion wild
wild pansy, *see* Johnny jump-up
wild peach, *see* peach, wild
wild strawberry, *see* strawberry, wild
willow, blue, 58
willow, gray, 28, 189, **190**
wintergreen, *see* wintermint

wintermint, **191**
witch grass, **191**
wood betony, **191–192**
wood rose, *see* rose, wood
woodwardia, 28
wormwood (mugwort), 13, 78, 81, 83,
   85, 86, 88, 102, 115, 122, 133,
   140, 162, 166, 172, **192–194**,
   199, 200
Wyethia spp., 152
xannáachyuh, 158
xanpúttin, 156
xánthiip, 156

Xanthium strumarium, 107
xáyviish, 154
xunyêep, 183
xunyêepshurukhitihan, 165
xuppáriish, 196
xutyúppin, 111
yarrow, 28, 81, 184, **194**
yellow dock, *see* dock, curly
yellow monkeyflower, *see*
   monkeyflower, yellow
yellow mustard, *see* mustard, yellow
yerba buena, 5, 13, 72, 75, 139, 151,
   152, 158, 159, **195**
yerba santa, *see* mountain balm
yew, **196**
yumaaréempeeshara, 191
Zea mays, 115
Zingiber officinalis, 127

acne, *see* skin diseases, acne
age spots, *see* skin diseases, spots
alcohol
    anti-intoxicant, 168
    cleanse from system, 192, 193
    decrease desire for, 101, 134
    effect on healing sores, 200
    hangover, 120
    withdrawal, 165
allergies
    asthma, *see* asthma
    hay fever, 153
    prevention, 162
    skin rash, *see* skin diseases, rash,
        allergic
Alzheimer disease, *see* memory loss
anemia, 118
angina, *see* heart, angina
appetite improvement, 103
arteries, clogged, *see* heart, clogged
    arteries
arteriosclerosis, *see* heart,
    arteriosclerosis
arthritis, 79, 101, 179, 181, 192, 193,
    197
asthma, 87, 88, 109, 111, 133, 135,
    152, 153, 195
back pain, 140, 143
bad breath, *see* mouth, bad breath
bedsores, *see* sores, bedsores
bed-wetting, *see* kidneys, bed-wetting
bee sting, *see* insects, bee sting
bile-secretion, *see* liver, bile-secretion
bite, insect, *see* insect bite
bite, spider, *see* spider bite
black eye, *see* eyes, black
bladder
    conditions, 115, 118, 141
    dissolves gravel, 130
    infection, 118, 153
    problems from bad kidneys, 165,
        191
    urination, difficult, 118
bleeding, *see* wounds
bleeding gums, *see* mouth, gums,
    bleeding
bleeding ulcers, *see* ulcers, bleeding
blisters
    fever, 105
    mouth, 109

mucous membrane, 109
    prevention of on skin, 81, 107
blood poisoning, 23, 80, 162, 163, 190
blood pressure, high, 74, 111, 114, 120,
    126, 127, 130, 154, 160, 183
    birth control, 142, 150
boils, external, 23, 79, 80, 86, 102, 113,
    114, 115, 118, 124, 153, 162,
    163, 166, 172, 180, 192, 193
    gum, 105, 169, 182
bowel, hemorrhage, *see* hemorrhage,
    bowel
broken limb, *see* limb, broken
bronchial trouble, *see* lungs, bronchial
    trouble
bronchitis, 88, 111, 133, 152, 153
bruise, *see* skin, bruises
burns,
    pain, 107
    prevention of blistering from,
        107,148
    radiation burns, 197
    treatment, 79, 148, 156, 157, 183
cancer, 129, 160, 161
    cancerous sores, *see* sores,
        cancerous
    external cancerous sores, *see*
        sores, external cancerous
    hold down food, 107, 132, 182
    internal, 113, 156, 196, 197
    mouth, 180
    prevention of some types, 124,
        190
    skin, 172, 192, 193
    swelling from cancer nodes, 120
    tumors, 106, 120
cankers, mouth, *see* mouth, cankers
canker sores, *see* sores, canker
carbuncles, 79, 80, 124, 167
cataracts, *see* eyes, cataracts
childbirth
    hemorrhage, 175
    labor pains, 114, 151, 178
    morning sickness, 121, 127, 160
    strengthening uterine wall, *see*
        uterine wall, strengthen
cholesterol, 101, 126
circulation, 79, 108, 114, 127, 131, 140
cleanser, liver, *see* liver, cleanser
cold, 75, 76, 81, 86, 96, 109, 138, 139,

    161, 162, 164, 170, 171, 177,
    188, 192, 193, 195
    phlegm, *see* phlegm
    prevention of, 76, 77, 78, 95, 96,
        126, 134, 135, 139, 160, 161,
        162, 163, 170, 192, 193, 195
    treating congestion from, 154, 155
    treating fever from, 124
colic, 76, 108, 139, 180, 181
colitis, 129, 162, 163, 164
congestion from smoke, *see* lungs,
    congestion, and phlegm
constipation, 124, 136,
convulsions, 108, 133, 142, 150, 161,
    162, *see also* fits
cough, 87, 88, 111, 133, 135, 146, 194
    phlegm, *see* phlegm
    whooping, 76, 133, 135, 152, 188,
        195
cramps
    feet, 186
    leg, 186
    menstrual, *see* menstrual, cramps
    stomach, 191
cut, *see* wound
diabetes, 103, 104, 108, 114, 117, 118,
    137, 142, 147, 170, 171
    diabetic feet, 79, 140, 192, 193
    diabetic sores, 23, 79, 81, 86, 162,
        163
    dropsy, 108, 108, 114, 117, 137,
        140, 141, 142, 147, 171
diarrhea, 126, 175, 189, *see also*
    bowel, hemorrhage
dropsy, *see* diabetes
drugs, 101
    cleanse from system, 192, 193
    drug babies, 77, 88, 152
    jaundice from, 191
    withdrawal, 165
dry hair, *see* hair, dry
dry skin, *see* skin diseases, dry
ear
    ache, 162, 163
    infection, 146, 164
eczema, *see* skin diseases, eczema
emphysema, *see* lungs, emphysema
epilepsy, 114, 142, 146, 150, 162, 176
eyes
    black, 181

cataracts, 80, 95, 122, 123, 156, 157, 183
  pink (sties), 116
  sore, 116
eyesight
  nutrition and, 122
  see also cataracts
fertility, 166
fever
  blisters, *see* blisters, fever
  breaking, 135, 141, 194
  prevention, 161, 195
  reduction, 122, 124, 140, 141, 151, 157, 167, 171–172, 184, 194
fingernails, loss *see* nails, loss
fish bone injuries, 162, 163
fits, 133, 160, 176, *see also* convulsions
fleas, *see* insects, fleas
flu
  fever reduction, 122,
  prevention, 77, 78, 87, 134, 159, 160, 162, 163, 195
  stomach, 148, 182
  treatment, 87, 119, 122, 159, 170, 195
flukes, in cows and horses, 102
food poisoning, 173, *see also* poisoning, food
freckles, *see* skin diseases, freckles
gallstone, 130, 149, 157
gas, 108, 126, 127, 138, 139, 162, 180, 181, *see also* indigestion, intestinal putrefaction and pain, gas
gingivitis, *see* mouth, gingivitis
goiters, 106, 174, 175
gout, 131, 171, 173
gums, bleeding, *see* mouth, bleeding gums
gum boils, *see* mouth, gum boils
hair
  dryness, 78–79, 122, 123, 124
  gray, 174, 189
  lice, *see* insects, lice
  loss, 131, 174, 188
hangover, *see* alcohol, hangover
hay fever, *see* allergies, hay fever
headache, 140, 141, 160, 161, 186
  migraine, 123
heart
  ailments, 108, 111, 120, 121, 132
  angina, 146
  arteriosclerosis, 120
  beat regulation, 111
  clogged arteries, 101

high blood pressure, *see* blood pressure, high
  pain, 111, 120
  weakness, 132, 146, 159
heartburn, 138
hemorrhage
  bowel, 153
  childbirth, *see* childbirth, hemorrhage
  lungs, 153
  ulcers, stomach, 180
HIV/AIDS, 161, 194
  cleansing system, 129, 132
  hold down food, 107
  settle stomach, 121, 182
hot flashes, 121
hunger, 95
hyperactivity, 130
hypoglycemia, 171
hysteria, 160
impetigo, *see* sores, impetigo
impotence, 117
indigestion, 127, 162, *see also* gas and stomach, sour
infection, *see* sores, infections, and wound
insects
  bee sting, 102, 170, 171
  bite, 102, 170, 171, 197
  fleas (on cats and dogs), 122
  lice, 122, 192, 193, 194
  mosquito bite, 170
  sting, 105, 170, 197
insomnia, 102, 108, 134, 136, 137, 165, 186, *see also* nerves and restlessness
intestine, 129, 132, *see also* colitis
intestinal putrefaction, 126
jaundice, 77, 103, 110, 135, 180, 191, 192, 193, *see also* HIV/AIDS, jaundice
kidneys, 109, 110, 115, 118, 153, 158, 159
  bed-wetting, 115
  failure, 152, 158, 195
  infections, 118, 153
  problems related to pancreas and adrenal glands, 141
  stones, 130, 149, 157, 188
  urination, difficult, 118
  urination, excessive, 180
  urination, painful, 115
  urine blockage, 109
  urine leakage, 109
lice, *see* insects, lice
limbs

broken bones, 178, 179
  bruises, *see* skin, bruises
  cramps, *see* cramps, feet and leg
  sensation loss, 117
  sprain, 79, 80, 119, 179, 192, 193
liver
  bile-secretion, 103
  cirrhosis, 152, 158, 159, 195
  cleanser, 111, 128, 129
  jaundice, 110
  kidney infections, relation to, 118
longevity, 136
lungs, 184
  bronchial trouble, 109
  bronchitis, *see* bronchitis
  congestion from smoke, 152, 153, 195
  emphysema, 109
  hay fever, *see* allergies, hay fever
  hemorrhage, *see* hemorrhage, lungs
  pneumonia, 109, 111
  strengthen, 101, 183
  tuberculosis, 101, 109, 155, 176, 184
  whooping cough, *see* cough, whooping
mange, *see* skin diseases, mange
memory loss, 130
menopause, 114, 160
menstruation
  cramps, 114, 127, 161
  excessive flow, 161
morning sickness, 121, 127, 160
mourning, 137
mouth
  bad breath, 155, 159, 177
  blistering, 109
  blisters, *see* blisters, mouth
  cancer, *see* cancer, mouth
  cankers, 105
  canker sores, 113, 169, 180, 181, 182, 190
  cold sores, 171
  fungus, 126, 127
  gingivitis, 101
  gum boils, 105, 169, 182
  sores, 105, 169, 170, 182
  sore throat, *see* sore throats
  strep throat, 78, 116, 126, 134, 170
  tonsillitis, 105, 125, 126, 155, 177, 192, 193
  ulcers, 169
mucous membrane blistering, *see* blisters, mucous membrane

muscle
      pain, 165
      sore, 179
      spasm, 186
      strengthen action of, 146
      twitching, 186
nails (finger and toe)
      loss, 174
      weak, 188
nausea from radiation therapy, 121
nerves, 108, 114, 165, 186, *see also*
            insomnia and restlessness
nosebleeds, 113
pain
      back pain, *see* back pain
      childbirth, *see* childbirth, labor
            pains
      diabetic feet, *see* diabetes, diabetic
            feet
      gas, 108, 162, 181, *see also* gas
      general, 84, 86, 187
      heart, *see* heart, pain
      muscle, *see* muscle, pain
      skin sores, 166
      sores that don't heal, 140, *see also*
            sores, that don't heal
      terminal illness, *see* terminal
            illness
      toothache, *see* toothache pain
      urination, painful, 115
      see also burns, pain
pancreatitis, 77, 158, 159
parasites (internal), 129, 132, 189, *see*
            also worms and skin diseases,
            ringworm
Parkinson's disease, 182, 191, 192
piles, 136, 166, 167
pink eye, *see* eyes, pink
pinworm, *see* worms, pinworm
pituitary gland, 101
pneumonia, *see*, lungs, pneumonia
poisoning
      food, 173
      mushroom, 173
      star thistle, 114
poison oak, 79–80, 81, 84, 118, 148,
            153, 166, 168, 178, 189, 192,
            193, 197
      preventative, 179
prostate, 115, 128, 141
psoriasis, *see* skin diseases, psoriasis
pyorrhea, *see* mouth, gum boils
reproductive organs, 117
restlessness, 134, 186, *see also*
            insomnia and nerves
rheumatism, 173, 190

ringworm, *see* skin diseases, ringworm
scabies, *see* skin diseases, scabies
sensation loss in limbs, *see* limbs,
            sensation loss
shingles, 162, 163, 164
sinus
      congestion, 163, 181
      infection, 162, 163
skin diseases, 79, 81, 86, 113, 114, 115,
            118, 140, 153, 166, 192, 193,
            197
      acne, 172, 192, 193
      arthritis, *see* arthritis
      blisters, *see* blisters
      boils, *see* boils, external
      bruise, 79, 113, 178, 181, 192, 193
      cancer, *see* cancer, skin
      dry, 84, 118, 153, 166
      eczema, 84, 118, 153, 166
      freckles, 116
      mange (on animals), 86, 115, 140,
            153, 166, 192, 193
      moles, pre-cancerous, 190
      pain, *see* pain, skin sores
      psoriasis, 79, 84, 86, 115, 118, 140,
            153, 166, 172, 173, 192, 193,
            197
      rash, 79, 169, 189
         allergic, 74, 166
         heat, 166
         poison oak, *see* poison oak
      ringworm, 86, 115, 140, 153, 166,
            192, 193
      scabies, 86, 115, 140, 153, 166,
            192, 193
      sores, *see* sores
      spots, 103, 118, 169
      sunburn, 84, 118, 153, 166
      warts, 118, 124, 149, 185
      yeast infections, 79, 80, 92,192,
            193
      see also wound
sores, 119
      bedsores, 23, 84, 114, 133, 140,
            162, 192, 193
      cancerous, external, 84, 114, 133,
            149, 192, 193, 200
      canker, *see* mouth, cankers
      diabetic, *see* diabetes, diabetic
            sores
      impetigo, 23, 86, 118, 153, 162,
            166, 167
      infection, 50, 79, 86, 118, 164,
            166, 179
      mouth, 105
      pain, *see* pain, skin sores

that don't heal, 86, 113, 114, 115,
            118, 120, 133, 140, 141, 153,
            166, 182, 190, 192, 193, 200
      ulcerated, 23, 84, 86, 113, 114,
            115, 118, 133, 140, 153, 166,
            192, 193, 199
sore throats, 78, 88, 105, 115, 125,
            129, 135, 155, 170, 174, 177,
            181, 182, 192, 193, 194
smoking, withdrawal, 165
snake bite, 162
sour stomach, *see* stomach, sour
spider bite, 102, 162
      black widow, 134, 163
      see also insects, bee sting, insects,
            bite, and insects, mosquito bite
spleen
      jaundice, 110, 136
sprains, *see* limbs, sprain
star thistle poisoning, see poisoning,
            star thistle
sties, *see* eye, pink
strep throat, *see* mouth, strep throat
stress, 146, *see also* relaxant
sting, bee, *see* insect, bee stings
sting, insect, *see* insect stings
stomach
      cramps, *see* cramps, stomach
      flu, *see* flu, stomach
      gas, *see*
      morning sickness, *see* childbirth,
            morning sickness
      sour, 138, 139, 180, 181, *see also* gas
      ulcers, *see* hemorrhage, stomach
            ulcers
      upset, 48, 107, 132, 170, 182
      see also HIV/AIDS, settle stomach
strep throat, 78, 116, 126, 134, 170
stroke, 80, 160, 162, 173, 181
sunburn, *see* skin diseases, sunburn
syrup, cough, *see* cough syrup
TB, *see* tuberculosis
terminal illness,146, 176
toenail loss, *see* nails, loss
tonsillitis, 78, 105, 125, 126, 155, 177,
            192, 193, 199
toothache, 163, 162, 165, 174, 185
tooth care, 102
tuberculosis, 101, 109, 176, 184
      preventative, 155
tumors, *see* cancer
typhoid, 103
ulcerated sores, *see* sores, ulcerated
ulcer
      bleeding, 108, 126, 129, 133, 173,
            175

intestinal, 162, 163
pain, 108
stomach, *see* hemorrhage, stomach
  ulcers
urine
  excessive urination, 180
  painful urination, 115
  urine leakage, 109
uterine wall, 105, 128
varicose veins, 131, 174
venereal disease (gonorrhea and
  syphilis), 151

warts, *see* skin diseases, warts
weak nails, *see* nails, weak
weight reduction, 174, 175, 180
whooping cough, *see* cough,
  whooping
worms, 189, 191
  hookworms, 126
  in dogs, 129, 191
  pinworms, 197
  see also parasites and skin
    diseases, ringworm

wounds, 164, 166, 169, 170, 173, 179
  infected, 179
yeast infections, *see* skin diseases,
  yeast infections

acorn, 21, 22, 28, 30, 31, 46, 72, 80, 93, **94–95**, 96, 97, 101, 107, 148, 156, 157, 183, 192
    basket, 93, 148
    biscuits and bread, 95
    flour, 72, 94, 97, 107, 156, 157, 183
    leaching, 93, 94, 95, 97, 157
    leaching water, 80, 156, 157, 183
    processing, 94–95
    soup, 46, 93, 94, 95, 96, 183
Alaska, 50, 119, 134
animals, *see* bear, deer, eels, elk, fish, salmon
aromatic steam, *see* steam, aromatic
bacon
    grease, 78, 97, 174
    poultice, 80
basketry, 12, 21, 46, 51, *see also* education
    baskets, 21, 22, 27, 34, 37, 43, 44, 46, 47, 53, 54, 55, 56, 58, 72, 88, 90, 93, 94, 96, 97, 148, 149, 156, 189
    basketweavers, 11, 13, 16, 28, 34, 46, 54, 56, 57, 58, 59, 60, 94, 172, 199
    burn upon death, 137
    camps, 60
    collections, 52
    cooking in, 35
    demonstrating, 52, 53, 54, 59, 62
    designs, 44, 47, 51, 55, 58
    dye, 28, 58, 170, 189, 193
    history, 51–61
    innovation, 56
    land management, 11–12, 30–32, 43, 56, 57, 199, *see also* Karuk, land management
    learning, 42–43, 46, 58
    materials, 28, 31, 32, 42–43, 56, 58, 125, 133, 156, 170, 177, 189, 190, *see also* beargrass
    organizations, 11, 12, 13, 16, 46, 59, 69, 199
    selling, 51, 53, 54–56, 61, 62
    teaching, 42–43, 46, 52, 56–60
    tourist industry, 34
bear
    black, 30, 31, 39, 90, 91, 92

grease (fat), 39, 92
    grizzly, 34
    meat, 30
beargrass, 10, 12, 30, 31, 56, 62
Bennett, George (maternal grandfather, 1877–1934), 38
Bennett, Louise Nelson (maternal grandmother, 1881–1966), 38, 90, 117, 157, 194
Bennett, Maggie, *see* Grant, Maggie Bennett
berries (for food), 89–93, 97, 104, 105, 112, 130, 137, 147, 148, 149, 172, 173, 182, 184, 186
blood purifier (herbal medicine), 71, 75, 76, **76–77**, 80, 104, 107, 110, 112, 119, 120, 121, 129, 133, 134, 138, 139, 150, 151, 155, 158, 159
Brazille, Ellen (paternal grandmother, 1856–1940), 15, 36, 48, 61, 66, 81, 82, 118, 130, 153, 157, 167, 199
Brazille, Francis (paternal great-grandfather), 34–36
Brazille, Frank, *see* Brazill, Francis
Brazille, Susan, 48, 61, 66
Brazille, Queen (paternal great-grandmother), 36, 37, 48
British Columbia, 50, 119, 128, 134, 136
burning, effects, *see* basketry, land management, and Karuk, land management
burning practices, *see* Karuk, land management
butter, 92, 93, 171, 199, *see also* fruit butters
California Indian Basketweavers Association, 13, 16, 46, 69, 199
Canada, 34, 49, 74, 123, 134, 155, 177
canning, 27, 28, 84, **91–92**, 104, 137, *see also* fruit, canning
    cherries, 28, 105
    jar, 75, 93, 175, 199
    pot, 79
    tomatoes, 98

capsule (herbal medicine), 80, 106, 107, 108, 112, 114, 129, 146, 162, 171, 172, 181, 189
chew (herbal medicine), 77, 78, 88, 101, 102, 105, 125, 133, 139, 159, 165, 169, 170, 174, 180, 182, 185
Chief Su-Worhom, *see* Risling, David, Sr.
childhood, *see* Josephine Peters, childhood
Chinese herbalists, *see* herbalists, Chinese, and Yen family
Chinese miners, 72, 123, 132, *see also* miners
chowchow, **98**
cleanser (herbal medicine), **77–78**, 80, 11, 80, 111, 129, 150, 168, 193
coffee, 110, 128
    can, 163
    cup, 75, 127
    grinder, 166
    pot, Pyrex, 82, 85, 86, 87, 145
Columbia, 49, 110
cordage, 139
cough drops (herbal medicine), 87, **88–89**
cough syrup (herbal medicine), *see* syrup
county fairs, *see* fairs, county and state
cultural proscriptions, *see also* Karuk, cultural proscriptions and spirituality
damage to gathering areas, *see* gathering, site damage
dangers of plant use, see plant use,
decoration (plant), 125
deer, 12, 30, 31, 35, 36, 46, 170
    grease, 149
    meat (venison), 28, 30, 78
diuretic (herbal medicine), 118, 151, 159, 169, 180, 188
douche (herbal medicine), 128, 181
drink, medicinal
    cold, 134, 136
    see also tea
drink, non-medicinal, *see* water, flavored
drops (herbal medicine)

cough, *see* cough drops
   ear, 162, 163
   from dropper, 76, 106, 118, 127,
      129, 163, 181, 195, 199
   nose, 181
drugs, 77, 88, 101, 129, 152, 165, 191,
      see also marijuana
drying and storing medicines, *see*
      medicines, herbal, drying and
      storing
dye
   basketry *see* basketry, dye
   hair, 189
eat (herbal medicine), 162, 163
education
   cultural, 42–43, 61–67, 139, *see*
      also basketry, teaching
   school, 39, 42, 43, 44, 48, 51, 52,
      59, 60, 62, 80, 108, 118, 138,
      144, 145, 153, 167, 194, 197
eels, 28, 30, 46, 104
   grease, 164
elk, 12
   meat, 28, 30, 46
emetic (herbal medicine), 146
enema (herbal medicine), 166, 167
entertainment, 41–42, 60, 106, 116,
      186, *see also* marathons
   games, 41, 42, 106, 116
   wrestling, 41, 101, 183
   see also Peters, Josephine,
      childhood
Epsom salt, 79, 167, *see also* soaks
eyewash (herbal medicine), 80, 94, 95,
      122, 156, 157, 174, 183, *see*
      also washes
fairs, county and state, 45, 50, 51,
      53–54, 57, 59, 61, 62
family history, *see* Josephine Peters,
      family history
first full moon in April, 16, 28, 71, 81,
      199
fish, 21, 27, 28, 46, 93, 98, 104, 162,
      163, *see also* salmon
flavoring,
   food, 126, 169, 190
   in mouth, 128, 144, 145, 152
   medicinal teas, 106, 112, 120, 127,
      129, 136, 144, 146, 162, 165,
      180, 181
   see also water, flavored
floods, 33, 42, 45, 52, 57, 146, 196
flour
   commercial, 81, 88, 92, 93, 154, 200
   acorn, *see* acorn flour
   mill, 93, 94, 166

sack, 75, 82, 87, 88, 90, 91, 94, 125
foods
   mushrooms, **93**
   native plants, **89–98**, *see* acorn,
      bacon, berries, chowchow,
      flour, fruit, grease, greens,
      fish, fruit, Indian bread,
      mushrooms, nuts, onion, non-
      native, pancakes, sourdough,
      pickle lily, salad, salsa, soup
   native animals, see bear, deer, eels,
      elk, fish, salmon
   other foods, **97–98**, see butter,
      fruit, salsa, tomatoes, pickle
      lily, chowwow, pancakes,
      sourdough
   seaweed, **96–97**
Forest Service, 12, 13, 30, 42, 56, 57,
      58, 64, *see also* national forest
Forks of Salmon, 33, 36, 38
fragrance
   candle (for repellent), 144
   hair, 144
fried pie, *see* fruit, pie, fried
fruit (native), 27, 28, 36, 39, 41, 78,
      79, **89–93**, 101, 102, 104, 105,
      109, 116, 117, 124, 130, 137,
      148, 167, 170, 175, 182
   butters, **97–98**
   canning, **91–92**, 93, 104, 137
   cooked, **91–93**, 102, 104, 117, 122
   duff, 92, 93, 102, 104, 137
   gooseberries, 90
   grape, non–native, 101, 105, 154
   huckleberries, 90
   jam, **91–92**, 102, 104, 105, 167
   jelly, **91–92**, 102, 104, 105, 117,
      137, 167, 172
   manzanita berries, 90
   pie, 90, 91, **92**, 102, 104, 105, 117,
      127, 130, 137
   pie, fried, **92**, 102, 104, 105, 137
   plum, 91
   plum, cherry, 91
   steam pudding, 93, 137
fry bread, *see* Indian bread
games, *see* entertainment, games
garden, 27, 28, 31, 39, 68, 72, 74, 126,
      138, 162, 169, 170, 190
gargle (herbal medicine), **78**, 105, 109,
      115, 125, 126, 127, 129, 135,
      155, 174, 177, 181, 182, 192,
      193, 194, 199
gathering cycle, *see* plant gathering,
      seasonality
Golden Metal Discovery, 113

grease (types), 35, 78, 95, 149, 164,
      174, 200
Grant, Hugh (paternal grandfather,
      1847–1924), 36–37, 185
Grant (Mrs. Frank), Maggie Bennett
      (mother), 37, 38, 39, 42, 45,
      56, 59, 79, 80, 83, 86, 89, 90,
      91, 92, 93, 97, 98, 105, 107,
      112, 124, 153, 155, 170, 190
Grant, Sr., Frank A. (father), 37,
      39–40, 48, 60, 79, 80, 83, 102,
      138, 167, 185
greens, 30, 169
   shoots, 104, 105,
   see also salad (ingredients)
gum
   licorice, 106
   milkweed, 60, 149
   pitch, 125
Hailstone, Vivien, 15, 23, 25, 51, 52,
      53, 54, 55, 56, 57, 58, 59
hair fragrance, *see* fragrance, herbal
harvesting plants, *see* plant gathering
herbalists, Chinese, 10, 48, 74, 101,
      123, 130, 132, 136, 144, 159,
      174
herbal medicines, *see* medicines,
      herbal
Hoopa Pottery Guild, *see* pottery,
      Hoopa Pottery Guild
Hoopa Valley, 16, 101, 108, 112, 132,
      134, 154, 169, 185, 186, 188
Indian bread, 200
inhalant (herbal medicine), **78**
insect repellent, *see* repellent, insect
I-Ye-Quee, 54, 55, 56
Johnson, Ella, 45, 47, 53, 54, 55, 56,
      57, 58, 59, 61, 63, 172
Jones, Flora, 95, 132, 161
Junction school, 39, 40, 42, 39, 40, *see*
      also education, schooling
Karuk
   cultural proscriptions, 21–22, 25,
      32, 48
   cultural renaissance, 51–65
   culture, 29–32
   history, 9, 10, 32–33
   homeland, 28–29
   land management, 10, 12, 30–32,
      43, 56, 57, 58, 64, 74, 91,
      see also basketry, land
      management
   material culture, 30
   political system, 30
   social system, 30
   spirituality, 21–22, 25, 29–30, 32, 48

values, 28, 32, 46, 47, 68
worldview, 21–22, 25, 29–30, 32
Karuk Indigenous Basketweavers, 11, 12
Klamath–Trinity Hoopa Basketweavers, 56, 59
Lady Pinkums, 113
Lagrave, Francis, *see* Brazill, Francis
lampreys, *see* eels
land management, *see* basketry, land management, and Karuk, land management
laxative (herbal medicine), 103, 109, 111
licorice gum, *see* gum, licorice
Maddux, Phoebe, 42, 43, 102
marathons, 101, 183, *see also* Redwood Empire Marathon
marijuana, 87, 88, 135, 152, 200
mask (cucumber facial), 116
mechanical (herbal medicine), 188
medicines, herbal, **71–89**
dangerous qualities, *see* plant use, dangerous plants, and plant use, dangers
drying and storing, **72**
types of, *see* blood purifier, capsule, chew, cleanser, cough syrup, diuretic, douche, drink (cold), drops (cough, from dropper, ear, and nose), eat, emetics, enema, eyewash, fragrance, gargle, inhalant, laxative, mask, mechanical, moisturizer, mouthwash, paste, penicillin, plaster, poultice, repellent, rinse, salve, sedative, soak, soap, steam (aromatic), suck, syrup, tattoo, tea (decoction), tonic, wad, wash
non-plant, 197, *see* oatmeal, ocean water, olive oil, Redmond clay, serpentine mud
testing, **74**
preparation, **74**
miners, 32–33, 36, 39, 86, *see also* Chinese miners and mining
mining, 32–33, 34, 35, 36, 38, 39–40, 86, 89, 123, 124, 131, 190, *see also* miners
moisturizer, 171
mosquito repellent, see repellent, mosquito
mouthwash (herbal medicine), 118, 155

mushrooms (food), 28, 69, 73, 93, 127, 147, 154
national forest, 11, 12, 13, 17, 69
native animal foods, *see* foods, native animal
native plant foods, *see* foods, native plants
New Mexico, 58, 59, 108
nuts (native plant), 23, 25, 30, 42, 50, 56, 77, 78, 81, 86, 89, **94–96**, 105, 109, 133, 134, 153, 157, 162–164, 183, 189, 190, 200
hazelnuts, 95
peppernuts, 95–96
pine nuts, 96
see also acorns
oatmeal (non-plant medicine), 197
ocean water (non-plant medicine), 168, 197
Old Home Place, 37, 38, 41, 43, 65, 86, 88, 89, 90, 91, 102, 112, 138, 149, 169, 189, 190, 197
olive oil (non-plant medicine), 50, 81, 84, 85, 86, 118, 163, 166, 197
onion, non-native, 86 (syrup), 93, 98, *see also* onion, wild
Oregon, 28, 36, 101, 103, 119, 127, 162, 196
pancakes, sourdough, **98**
paste (herbal medicine), **81**, 102, 148, 156, 157, 190
penicillin (herbal medicine), 179
Peters, Josephine
childhood, 39–44
family history, 33–38
maternal family history, 38
paternal family history, 34–37
herbalism, 48–51, 65
homelife, 27–28
motherhood, 45–48
plant knowledge, 10, 48–50, 74, 105, 108, 109, 110, 111, 112, 113, 116, 118, 119,121, 122, 123, 124, 125, 126, 129, 130, 131, 132, 134, 135, 136, 141, 142, 143, 146, 147, 150, 159, 174
Red Wing Indian Handcrafts, 60–61
teaching, 61–65
travels (in other states and countries), 49, 59, 62, 74, 106, 129, 146, 174, *see also* Alaska, British Columbia, Canada, Columbia, New Mexico, Oregon, South America,

Vermont
phlegm, 188
pickle lily, **98**
pie, *see* fruit, pie
pine
pine nut beads, 96
pine nuts, 30, 56, 96
pitch, 78, 88, 96
plant gathering, **71–72**
damage, including from overharvesting, 9, 13, 114, 128, 138, 154, 155, 176, 186
ethics, 9, **67–69**
horticultural techniques, *see* Karuk, land management
land management, *see* Karuk, land management
seasonality, 12, 28, 32
spirituality, 32, 48, 68
techniques, 71–72
plant use, *see* foods and medicines, herbal
dangerous plants, 9, 48, 76, 108, 111, 114, 120, 141, 146, 150, 155, 160, 168, 174, 176, 183, 186, 187, 194
dangers, 13, 64, 72, 74, 75, 90, 101, 124, 141, 142, 150, 161, 188, 200
drying and storing, **72**
non-native plants, 72–73
poisonous plants, 48, 142, 150, 160
spirituality, 9, 32, 50, 74
plaster (herbal medicine), **81**, 154, 163
potato, non-native, 80. 126, 158, 159, *see also* Indian potato
pottery, 51, 52, 53, 54
designs, 51, 52, 55
Hoopa Pottery Guild, 51–53
Pottery Guild, Hoopa, *see* Hoopa Pottery Guiid
poultice (herbal medicine), 50, **80–81**, 86, 103, 107, 113, 114, 116, 119, 120, 124, 131, 148, 149, 153, 154, 156, 157, 163, 164, 166, 167, 169, 172, 173, 174, 180, 181, 183, 190, 192, 193, 194, 200
Raleigh man, 27, 113, 143, 154
Redmond clay (non-plant medicine), 197
Redwood Empire Marathon, 101, *see also* marathons
repellent (plant medicine)
fleas, 122

insect, 144, 186, 187
  mosquito, 144
  tick, 192, 193
rinse (herbal medicine)
  body, 193
  hair, **78–79**, 122, 123, 124, 192, 193
  mouth, 126, 127, 181, 199
Risling, David, Sr., 53, 54
salad (ingredients), 77, 103, 110, 150, 154, 159, 169, 180, 190
salmon, 28, 30, 46
  cooked, 28, 164
  eggs, 146
  grease (fat), 149
Salmon River, 30, 33, 36, 38, 39, 169
salsa, **98**
salve (herbal medicine), 28, 50–51, 72, 76, 79–80, **81–86**, 113, 114, 115, 118, 133, 134, 140, 141, 153, 166, 167, 172, 173, 192, 193, 194, 199
seasonality, *see* plant gathering, seasonality
sedative (herbal medicine), 154, 160, 178
serpentine mud (non-plant medicine), 197
  soil, 42, 146, 158, 176
soak (herbal medicine), **79**, 81, 114, 141, 153, 171, 192, 193, 194
soap (herbal medicine), 79, 177
soup, 103, 139, 154, 158, *see also*

acorn soup
South America, 49, 103
spirituality, 9, 50, *see also* Karuk, cultural proscriptions and spirituality
  in prescribing and using herbal medicines, 74, *see also* plant gathering and plant use, spirituality
steam, aromatic (herbal medicine), 162
stew, 98, 103, 138, 139, 158, 159
suck (herbal medicine), 128, 151, 178, 181
Sudden Oak Death, 68
Su-Worhom, Chief, *see* Risling, David, Sr.
syrup (herbal medicine), **86–88**, 89, 111, 133, 134, 135, 152, 195, 200
tattooing (herbal medicine), 168
tea, *see also* drink, medicinal, cold
  medicinal, 80, 101, 102, 103, 104, 107, 108, 109, 110, 111, 112, 113, 115, 117, 118, 119, 120, 121, 122, 123, 124, 126, 127, 128, 130, 132, 133, 135, 136, 137, 140, 141, 142, 143, 146, 147, 148, 150, 151, 152, 153, 155, 156, 157, 158, 160, 161, 162, 165, 166, 170, 171, 172, 173, 176, 180, 181, 182, 183,

184, 186, 187, 188, 190, 191, 192, 193, 194, 195, 196
  preparation, 72, **74–76**, 77
  non-medicinal, 75, 143, 162, 195
tick repellent, see repellent, tick
tomatoes, 91, **98**
tonic (herbal medicine), 136, 200, *see also* syrup
Traditional Medicine Program (Hoopa Valley), 49–50
types of herbal medicines, *see* medicines, herbal, types of
uncles, 28, 41, 44, 102, 159, 163, 164, 168, 173
vegetables, 27, 28, 36, *see also* greens
venison, *see* deer meat
Vermont, 106, 174
vitamins, 102, 107, 159, 170
wad (herbal medicine), 159, 163, 174, 185
wash (herbal medicine), **79–80**, 140, 141, 148, 153, 163, 166, 167, 189, 192, 193, *see also* eyewash and mouthwash
water, flavored, 90, 106, 143, 144, 145, 148, 149, 152, 165
Wistar, Issac J., 34–36
World War II, 44, 45, 53, 111
Yen family, 48, 74, 130, 136, 143, 159

About Beverly Oritz

Beverly R. Ortiz, Ph.D., is a lecturer in the anthropology
department at California State University East Bay,
contributing editor to "News from Native California",
ethnographic consultant and park naturalist.